THE CLINICAL COMPANION OF THE DONKEY

Produced by
The Donkey Sanctuary

Edited by
Linda Evans BVetMed MRCVS
Michael Crane BVM&S PGCE MRCVS

Matador
9 Priory Business Park,
Wistow Road, Kibworth Beauchamp,
Leicestershire. LE8 0RX
Tel: 0116 279 2299
Email: books@troubador.co.uk
Web: www.troubador.co.uk/matador
Twitter: @matadorbooks

The Donkey Sanctuary
Sidmouth, Devon, EX10 0NU
A charity registered with the Charity Commission for England and Wales.
No. 264818
Tel: 01395 578222
Email: vets@thedonkeysanctuary.org.uk
Email: research@thedonkeysanctuary.org.uk
Web: thedonkeysanctuary.org.uk

ISBN 978 1789013 900

British Library Cataloguing in Publication Data.
A catalogue record for this book is available from the British Library.

Printed and bound by CPI Group (UK) Ltd, Croydon, CR0 4YY

Matador is an imprint of Troubador Publishing Ltd

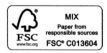

Dedicated to the memory of
Dr Elisabeth D. Svendsen MBE.
and to the continuing path at
The Donkey Sanctuary for improving
the health and welfare of donkeys worldwide.

ACKNOWLEDGMENTS

All the contributors to this handbook are employed by, or associated with, The Donkey Sanctuary and information is evidence based or is the shared experience of past and present members of staff. The content reflects this vast experience and knowledge and we would like to acknowledge and thank all the professions for their willingness to share information and findings for the greater good of the health and welfare of donkeys.

Special thanks must go to Neil Frame BVM&S CertEP CertVA MRCVS; RCVS Advanced Practitioner (Equine Practice) of Frame, Swift and Partners, Penrith. He has been enthusiastic in giving his time and experience to proof read and to provide the practical guidance on the relevance of the contents of this book to the practitioner and other professionals. His pertinent comments and advice have been valuable in ensuring this is a clear and easy reference tool for all those working with, or with an interest, in the health and welfare of donkeys.

We would also like to thank our proof readers, who have given their time and been thorough in making this the professional book that we aspired to; Alison Hills, freelance proof reader, New Zealand and Liz Hazell-Smith, Research Assistant at The Donkey Sanctuary.

No book would be complete without images and illustrations and we have used a comprehensive selection for reference. Kate Selley holds and manages a vast collection for The Donkey Sanctuary and she has used her drive, enthusiasm and positivity to obtain specific images for this book and also to select appropriate images from her collection. Her contribution to the book is much appreciated.

This book has been organised into systems in order to make reference quick and easy.

We have not included information about procedures or conditions for donkeys where they do not differ from those in horses and ponies, as there are already many excellent texts that describe these. Therefore, we have not included chapters on the Cardiovascular System, the Urinary System or Ophthalmology as we do not have any additional clinically relevant information that is specific to donkeys.

Each chapter contains specific information on the clinical examination and procedures as well as the common conditions for that system and we have used signposting to indicate where other chapters may contain additional useful information.

We do advise you to read the chapter on behaviour as this provides an explanation to the messages repeated throughout the book and is essential to your understanding of this unique animal.

TABLE OF CONTENTS

APPENDICES

FOREWORD

I first met the late Dr Elizabeth (Betty) Svendsen MBE, founder of The Donkey Sanctuary, in the mid 1970's. At that time Glasgow Veterinary School had an equine parasite research programme which included studies on equine lungworm infection. As donkeys were frequently infected with this parasite Dr Svendsen travelled north to find the best way to deal with the problem. This led to close collaboration between myself and The Donkey Sanctuary and resulted in Betty and I becoming good friends. Since then I have seen significant advances in knowledge of health and welfare of donkeys largely due to the efforts of their charismatic champion.

This latest Donkey Sanctuary publication "The Clinical Companion for the Donkey" would have pleased Betty enormously. It is a real Vade Mecum for everyone involved with donkeys to have by their side whether it be in developing countries where the donkey is a vital part of rural economies, or in parts of the world where they are kept either as pets or for leisure pursuits. Although much of the information provided in The Clinical Companion is relevant to donkeys worldwide some problems may be more important in certain areas - for example in Ethiopia it would be unusual to find an overweight laminitic donkey which, sadly, is not the case in many parts of Europe.

The Clinical Companion begins with an excellent chapter on donkey behaviour the understanding of which is fundamental for the detection of welfare or health problems.

I hope this valuable publication will be available to all who are involved with donkeys wherever they are and whatever their role.

James L Duncan BVMS PhD MRCVS
Professor Emeritus
The University of Glasgow

CONTRIBUTORS

Alex Thiemann MA Vet MB CertEP MSc CertVEd MRCVS

Senior Veterinary Surgeon- Education and Research at The Donkey Sanctuary.

Qualified from University of Cambridge (1989). Worked in mixed and then equine practice. Was a donkey owner as a child and joined the The Donkey Sanctuary in 1998. Gained Certificate in Equine Practice in 1995, Masters in International Animal Health in 2009 and Associate Fellowship of the Higher Education Authority in 2015. Has extensive donkey medical and surgical experience in the UK, Europe and with working donkeys globally. Has published numerous articles and contributions to books regarding donkey health and welfare.

Anna Haines BSc MSc

Lead in Behaviour in the Research and Operational Support Department at The Donkey Sanctuary.

Qualified from Liverpool University in Animal Behaviour (2004) and gained a Masters in Applied Animal Behaviour and Welfare (specialising in equines) in 2011. She has spent her career working for and managing a variety of equine and animal welfare charities internationally as well as in the UK and has worked as an equine behaviour consultant since 2012. Is a member of the 'Ask the Experts' team at Horse and Rider magazine and writes monthly feature articles for them and is a committee member for the Equine Behaviour and Training Association.

Anna Harrison BVSc BSc CertWEL MSc IAWEL AFHEA MRCVS

Veterinary Surgeon at The Donkey Sanctuary.

Qualified from University of Bristol (1986). Worked in mixed practice before joining Defra as a Veterinary Officer specialising in livestock welfare. Joined The Donkey Sanctuary in 2010. Gained Certificate in Animal Welfare Science, Ethics and Law in 1996, a Masters in International Animal Welfare, Ethics and Law in 2016 and Associate Fellowship of the Higher Education Authority in 2017 and is a RCVS Advanced Practitioner in Animal Welfare Science, Ethics and Law. Has worked abroad for equine and companion animal charities on a voluntary basis. Particular interests include all aspects of animal welfare and husbandry.

Ben Hart

Donkey Behaviour Training Manager at The Donkey Sanctuary.

A Certified Horse Behavioural Consultant (CHBC), registered with International Association of Animal Behaviour Councillors (IAABC) and a ABTC Registered Accredited Animal Behaviourist. Worked in America, Australia, Canada and Europe as an equine trainer, using the science of behaviour for training horses, donkeys and mules and to enhance the communication between animals and humans. His work is based around an understanding of the workings of the equine mind and use of positive reinforcement to motivate and encourage good behaviour in the animals with which he works.

Chris Garrett

Lead in Harnesses in the Research and Operational Support department at The Donkey Sanctuary.

Became a Master Harness Maker, Saddler and registered saddle fitter with a business in Shropshire. He taught challenged youngsters in Walsall, and was a registered ABW (carriage driver) for the Riding for the Disabled Association. Began working internationally in 2000 for an equine charity as an independent harness trainer and joined The Donkey Sanctuary in 2008. Travels extensively to countries where donkeys and mules are relied on for power; adapting harness from local materials, training owners and others concerned with improving the welfare of these animals, increasing efficiency and reducing harness related wounds. Interested in all traditional crafts and techniques.

Chris Platts BSc RSciTech

Laboratory Manager, at The Donkey Sanctuary.

Qualified from Bournemouth University with a degree in Forensic Sciences (2011). Joined The Donkey Sanctuary as a Laboratory Technician after graduating. A registered science technician and a member of The Royal Society of Biology. Delivers an efficient and bespoke service to The Donkey Sanctuary's veterinary and welfare teams.

Daniel Bacellar DVM

A clinician at AEPGA (Association for the Study and Protection of Donkeys). Qualified from the University of Évora in Portugal (2013). Works on welfare interventions involving education, general veterinary practice and dentistry and is also involved in breeding and stud management of the endangered Miranda Donkey Portuguese breed.

Elena Barrio MVDr Cert AVP MRCVS

Veterinary Surgeon at The Donkey Sanctuary.

Qualified from the University of Zaragoza in Spain (2003). Completed an externship in an Equine clinic in the UK and an internship in an Equine Hospital in Seville gaining experience in internal medicine and reproduction. Joined The Donkey Sanctuary in 2005, with responsibility for the new intake reception farm and the admissions of donkeys. Gained a Cert AVP in 2012 and currently working towards a PhD in Equine Veterinary Medicine.

Faith Burden BSc PhD

Director of Research and Operational Support at The Donkey Sanctuary.

Qualified from University of Warwick. Oversees The Donkey Sanctuary's research and technical services and has published over 50 peer reviewed articles relating to donkey health and welfare. Has a particular interest in donkey nutrition and parasitology and enjoys transforming scientific findings into evidence based practices for donkey owners and service providers globally.

Gemma Lilly BAEDT BSc(EDS) BA ESBM

Equine Dental Technician at The Donkey Sanctuary.

Qualified from West of England University with first class honours in Equine Dental Science (2005). Worked privately with working horses before joining The Donkey Sanctuary in 2007. Joined the Council for the British Association of Equine Dental Technicians in 2010, becoming chair in 2012. She formed part of the consortium developing the National Occupational Standards framework for equine dentistry in the UK. A regular lecturer, tutor and practical assessor in equine dentistry worldwide, Gemma became part of the examining board for the BEVA/BVDA examination for Equine Dental Technicians. Has published articles and contributed to books on equine dentistry and is known as an expert in the field of welfare oriented donkey and mule dentistry in the UK.

George Paraschou DVM MRCVS

Veterinary Pathologist at The Donkey Sanctuary.

Qualified from Aristotle University of Thessaloniki (2009). Completed an internship in equine medicine and surgery and carried out duties as a veterinary surgeon for the Greek Army before moving to the UK to work for the government at APHA. Was a donkey owner as a child and carried out voluntary work with donkeys for the Greek Animal Welfare Fund. Joined The Donkey Sanctuary in 2015 to work as a veterinary pathologist. Associate member of the Royal College of Pathologists.

Getachew Mulugeta DVM MVM PhD

Lead in Research in the Research and Operational Support department at The Donkey Sanctuary.

Qualified from Addis Ababa University (1992). Worked for the French Veterinary Mission and The International Livestock Research Institute before joining the Donkey Health and Welfare Project in Ethiopia. Returned to Addis Ababa University to work as a project leader and lecturer. Gained a Masters at Glasgow University followed by a PhD.

Jesus Buil MVDr MRCVS

Veterinary Surgeon at The Donkey Sanctuary.

Qualified from University of Zaragoza in Spain (2009). Completed an internship in equine medicine and surgery at the University of Zaragoza. Gained a Masters in 2011. Worked as a donkey clinician with working donkeys in Portuguese rural areas with AEPGA (Association for the Study and Protection of Donkeys) and in one of The Donkey Sanctuary holding bases in Portugal, focussing on orthopaedic conditions in the feet of the donkey. Joined The Donkey Sanctuary in 2016.

Jo Goliszek BVSc PGCert MRCVS

Veterinary Surgeon at The Donkey Sanctuary

Qualified from University of Bristol University (2011). Volunteered at a Veterinary clinic for working horses and donkeys in Egypt before doing an equine internship. Worked in equine practices before joining The Donkey Sanctuary in 2016. Interested in Animal Behaviour, Welfare and Internal Medicine.

João B. Rodrigues DVM PhD

Lead in Welfare in the Research and Operational Support department at The Donkey Sanctuary.

Qualified at University of Trás-os-Montes and Alto Douro (2007), classified as an Expert in Veterinary Dentistry and Maxillofacial Surgery by the Complutense University of Madrid (2011) and obtained a PhD focusing on research in the field of donkey dentistry (2013). Appointed as Professor of Medicine and Surgery of Equids in Portugal in 2013 and joined The Donkey Sanctuary in 2016. Has extensive donkey medical and welfare experience in Europe and with working donkeys globally, is a regular lecturer, tutor and practical assessor in equid dentistry worldwide and has published numerous articles and contributions to books. A former partner and board member of the Portuguese Association of Animal Traction (APTRAN).

Karen Pickering BVSc CertAVP(ED) PgCert VPS MRCVS

Veterinary Surgeon at The Donkey Sanctuary.

Qualified from the University of Bristol (2008). Worked in mixed practice before moving to The Donkey Sanctuary in 2010. Completed a Certificate in Advanced Veterinary Practice (Equine Dentistry) in 2017. Interests include dentistry and surgery. Has worked for equine charities overseas as a volunteer.

Karen Rickards BVSc PhD MRCVS

Head of Veterinary Services at The Donkey Sanctuary.

Qualified from University of Bristol (1994) and worked in equine practice for 4 years before undertaking a PhD in equine allergic airway disease at The Royal Veterinary College. Carried on working in this field as a post doc before taking up a lectureship in pharmacology at King's College, London. Started working at The Donkey Sanctuary in 2007. Main interest has always been lower airway inflammatory disease and the pharmacology of inflammation. Since working at The Donkey Sanctuary a new area of interest is pain recognition and its management in donkeys.

Miguel Quaresma DVM PhD

Clinician at the Veterinary Teaching Hospital and a researcher at CECAV, University of Trás-os-Montes and Alto Douro (UTAD).

Qualified at University of Trás-os-Montes and Alto Douro (1998) and obtained a PhD in Veterinary Sciences with the Thesis "Asinina de Miranda donkey breed (Equus asinus): demographic analysis and characterisation of the reproductive cycles." (2015). He has been working with donkeys since 2003, in collaboration with AEPGA.

Miguel Nóvoa DVM

Technical Secretary of the Miranda Donkey Portuguese breed since 2004 and responsible for the conservation and improvement programme of the breed.

Qualified at the University of Trás-os-Montes and Alto Douro (UTAD) (2003). Works on the animal welfare education campaign in rural areas of Portugal. A board member of the association AEPGA (Association for the Study and Protection of Donkeys) since 2002 and the association PALOMBAR since 2003.

Sue Dabinett

Head Veterinary Nurse at The Donkey Sanctuary.

Spent 5 years working in equine and small animal practice before joining The Donkey Sanctuary in 1982.

Rebekah Sullivan BVSc CertAVP(EM) MRCVS

Veterinary Surgeon at The Donkey Sanctuary.

Qualified from University of Bristol (2005). Worked in mixed practice and carried out periods of voluntary work abroad (Egypt and Morocco) with working equines. Joined The Donkey Sanctuary in 2012 and has been a member of the veterinary team ever since. Completed a certificate in equine medicine and is interested in most areas of veterinary medicine and surgery but is particularly keen on medical cases.

Vicky Grove BVSc MRCVS

Veterinary Surgeon at The Donkey Sanctuary.

Qualified from University of Liverpool (1996). Joined The Donkey Sanctuary in 1999. Qualified in acupuncture with a special interest in musculoskeletal conditions. Interested in surgery and anaesthesia.

Photographs and images

The majority of images in this handbook have been taken from the extensive libraries held at The Donkey Sanctuary, as well as from the private collections of the contributors.

The libraries held at The Donkey Sanctuary have been built by previous as well as present staff and contain a valuable resource for educational and training material.

The library of pathology images contains over 10,000 macroscopic and microscopic photographs of significant pathological findings identified over the past 15 years. George Paraschou and Chris Platts are currently managing the pathology laboratory archive of images.

The library of clinical work and research is managed by Kate Selley. She has over 12,000 images which are available as resources for education and training.

The images of dental conditions are from the private libraries belonging to João B. Rodrigues and Gemma Lilly and are part of an extensive collection covering all dental disorders in the donkey. Images belonging to Lee Gosden and Allan Emmett are also included.

INTRODUCTION

The Donkey Sanctuary has a mission: 'To transform the quality of life for donkeys, mules and people worldwide through greater understanding, collaboration and support, and by promoting lasting, mutually life-enhancing relationships.'

The Clinical Companion for the Donkey follows on from The Professional Handbook of the Donkey, which has been widely used as the definitive text for donkey medicine and surgery for many years. It is an updated and re-designed handbook which has been produced for clinicians and other professionals globally. Its aim is to improve the health, welfare and treatment of donkeys worldwide by providing easy reference and comprehensive guidance on the clinical care of donkeys. It enables us to share the vast expertise and experience of those working for, or associated with, The Donkey Sanctuary. In sharing this knowledge we believe that we play a part in educating and training those responsible for the management and clinical care of donkeys, therefore improving the quality of life of donkeys globally.

This book concentrates on the differences that are specific to donkeys. There are many excellent texts covering all the aspects of health and welfare of horses and ponies and this book has no intention of duplicating other work. Therefore, although the book has been organised in systems, there are some that have no additional donkey specific information and they are not covered. We have only included evidence based information or that of which we have significant experience at The Donkey Sanctuary. We have tried to cover global issues but it is important to take account of local legislation and regulations as well as available resources when referring to this book.

We have included a chapter on the behaviour of the donkey and feel that these principles explain the specific behaviour unique to this species and that this is a good introduction to handling, understanding and examining the donkey.

There are important messages and points to note when dealing with donkeys specifically, and to make this book a valuable and easy reference we have used highlighted boxes and signposts to draw attention quickly to those points, especially when in the field or faced with an emergency.

Images used in this book have been taken from the extensive libraries held at The Donkey Sanctuary, and belonging to contributors to the book.

There is limited knowledge of mules and hinnies and we have included what is known in tables at the end of each section.

The contents of this book and additional information are available to download from our website at:

thedonkeysanctuary.org.uk/for-professionals

The appendices are available as easy reference cards.

The website will be updated as and when new information or research becomes available and you are invited to sign up for news feeds of updates.

Lastly we have produced a book that we are proud of, with multiple authors covering a vast area of expertise and experience. We hope that this is a valuable reference tool for all those working with donkeys globally.

1. BEHAVIOUR

A knowledge and understanding of the unique characteristics of a donkey is valuable when handling, examining or carrying out a procedure.

The term 'stoic' is often used to describe donkey behaviour and we use it in relation to donkey behaviour throughout this book. Stoicism is typical predator-avoidance behaviour in a prey species such as the donkey; appearing strong and normal reduces the chances of a predator picking on you. This stoicity does not lessen the donkey's ability to experience pain and distress.

The donkey's behaviour is different from that of horses and ponies and it is crucial that this is taken into account when examining or attempting to carry out procedures. Their stoic nature serves them well but can lead to missing or misdiagnosing the severity of painful conditions. Their behaviour is often incorrectly labelled as stubborn, but a more accurate explanation for their behaviour is likely to be their sense of self-preservation. Using the correct behavioural principles and taking extra time will pay long term dividends when treating donkeys and mules.

The donkey is unlikely to show the dramatic signs of pain and distress exhibited by the horse and pony, even though it may be experiencing the same degree of pain.

BEHAVIOURAL TRAITS

RESTRAINT TECHNIQUES FOR PROCEDURES AND TREATMENT

COMMON BEHAVIOURAL PROBLEMS

KEY POINTS

- Donkeys are highly intelligent and capable of learning.

- Donkeys are extremely stoic, and subtle behavioural changes can indicate severe disease.

- Donkeys show subtle 'flight' responses and may 'freeze' or show 'fight' behaviours more readily than horses and ponies.

- If a nervous donkey shows symptoms of 'fight' behaviour, it is advisable to withdraw where possible and carry out a programme of retraining.

- Donkeys form strong pair bonds and the death of one donkey can result in stress induced hyperlipaemia in the companion.

The donkey has evolved to live in an environment with a sparse food supply and limited access to water. The behavioural repertoire of the donkey has enabled this species to thrive in these conditions and renders their behaviour significantly different from that of horses and ponies.

In an environment with limited natural resources, donkeys will graze and browse on forage with low nutritional value for 14—18 hours per day, regularly walking distances of 20—30km in 24 hours. Due to the sparsity of resources, donkeys do not have a tendency to form the large herds more typical of other equines, instead forming small groups or pairs, or even living solitary lives, searching for food and water and only coming together to breed or when environmental resources are plentiful.

Sexual behaviour is often more exaggerated in the donkey than in horses and ponies. Female donkeys are often seen to be cycling throughout the winter months, and stallion-like behaviour can persist strongly after stallions are castrated.

⚠ ALERT

Stallion-like behaviour is exaggerated and can persist after castration, therefore it is recommended that colt foals are castrated between 6 and 18 months.

Donkeys have both 'flight' and 'fight' instincts. Because they often live in pairs, small groups or on their own, fleeing is often not the best defence mechanism. **Fight behaviours are therefore more strongly established.** This can lead to conflict between donkeys and other domestic animals and be an issue with handling.

Despite the solitary life seen in resource limited environments, most domestic donkeys prefer to form pair bonds with members of the same species. However, they will occasionally form a strong bond with horses, ponies, mules or other species, despite having access to other donkeys.

> ⚠ **ALERT**
>
> Due to the formation of strong pair bonds, donkeys can suffer significant stress when their companion is removed, dies or is euthanased.

Vocalisation in the donkey includes their signature 'bray', which is unique to each individual donkey. The bray can travel over several kilometres. The stallion will use it to affirm their status. All donkeys use it to attract a mate, when isolated from their social group, or in anticipation of food. The donkey's ear position helps define the purpose of the bray:

- The ears are positioned gently backwards when greeting another donkey.

- Assertive animals hold their ears flat back when dealing with a threat.

- The ears are held firmly forward during sexual advances.

Donkeys may also learn to bray in anticipation of human activity such as feeding or attention from handlers.

BEHAVIOURAL TRAITS

The donkey is a stoic animal and rarely displays readily visible signs of pain, distress or fear. This makes inspection difficult and illness, pain and even severe conditions may be missed.

> ⚠ **ALERT**
>
> The dull or unusually quiet donkey should be regarded as a veterinary emergency.

It is vital to understand the behaviour of the donkey in order to recognise subtle changes that may indicate serious illness that requires immediate attention.

➜ *See Chapter 12: The Approach to the Dull Donkey for more information.*

Fear

Fear in the donkey may induce both 'flight' and 'fight' responses.

> ⚠ **ALERT**
>
> Signs of fear and stress may be subtle and easily overlooked.

Flight responses may be subtle and include:

- turning the head away from the handler
- stepping sideways slowly to avoid being caught
- 'freezing' in the presence of a fearful situation.

Fight responses can be a health and safety risk to both the animals and people and may include:

- Stamping, pawing and striking out
- head tossing
- biting
- leaning or pushing into the handler (dangerous when the handler is against a solid object)
- kicking out.

Donkeys can be very effective when kicking forwards with their hind legs. They can manage to make contact with a handler who is examining a forelimb.

Both responses increase stress levels and a concomitant risk of hyperlipaemia. Recognition of these responses will allow intervention to remove or limit any factors causing fear in the individual at an early stage.

It is possible to recognise facial expressions which will indicate fear in the donkey and these will allow early intervention.

The differences in facial expressions of a relaxed donkey compared to that same donkey exhibiting signs of fear/stress/anxiety.

Relaxed facial expressions		Facial expressions associated with fear/stress	
Relaxed, open nostrils	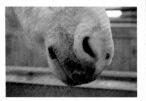	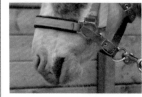	Nostrils clamped tightly shut
Relaxed muzzle – no visible wrinkles	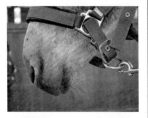	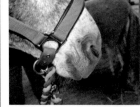	Tension around mouth leading to wrinkles forming around nostril and lips
Relaxed nostrils, even in shape	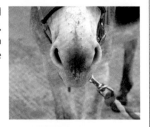	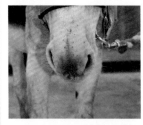	Uneven nostrils due to facial tension on right hand side leading to right nostril being drawn upwards
Eyes open, muzzle relaxed	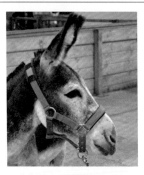	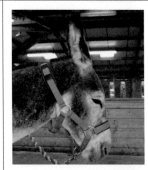	Eyes semi-closed with tense muzzle
Sclera not visible (care in some donkeys with sclera visible due to eye conformation)	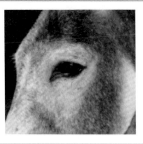	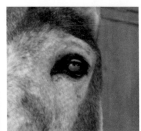	Palpebral fissure widened, sclera visible

It is often tempting to continue to attempt the procedure even when the donkey demonstrates fight behaviours. However, the situation can become dangerous and it is advisable to withdraw and reconsider the need for immediate intervention:

- The health and safety of the handler can become seriously compromised.

- The long term memory could make handling the donkey dangerous in the future.

- Results from any blood samples taken may be affected by stress levels.

- Any sedation or anaesthetic may be compromised.

⚠ ALERT

Experiences and fear learned during a procedure will affect future behaviour.

Gradual desensitisation, counter-conditioning and appropriate shaping plans can be used successfully for many problems, including the 'needle-shy' patient, and will lead to a safer and less stressed animal for future procedures.

Grief

Due to the formation of strong pair bonds, donkeys may suffer significant stress when their companion is removed, dies or is euthanased.

⚠ ALERT

The death or removal of a bonded companion may lead to severe stress, and subsequent anorexia and hyperlipaemia.

If euthanasia is expected or planned, it is worth considering the effect of companion loss on the survivor and making appropriate plans to reduce any stress.

See Chapter 15: Euthanasia and the Post-Mortem Examination for more information.

If it is appropriate for all the animals involved, another quiet donkey could be introduced over a fence to the pair prior to euthanasia. This will mean that the survivor is left with a companion within its visual field. After the euthanasia, a structured introduction can then be made between this pair.

The behavioural reaction to a euthanased companion can vary widely. It is recommended that when one of a pair bond dies, the companion is allowed to see and spend time with the dead body. Owners should be prepared to leave the pair together for as long as it takes for the companion to become disinterested in the body.

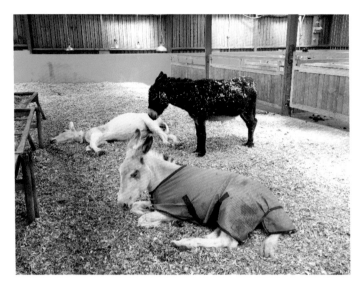

*Two donkeys'
response to
their euthanased
companion; each
lay down in turn
with the dead body
and remained in
her presence for
over an hour.*

The remaining donkey should be monitored carefully after the bereavement, paying special attention to appetite and feeding behaviour in order to minimise the risk of hyperlipaemia.

➔ *See Chapter 7: Hyperlipaemia and the Endocrine System for more information.*

If the survivor is left on its own after the bereavement, the need for a new companion should be assessed. Some animals will require another donkey almost immediately while others may appear to cope well on their own.

Stubborn behaviour

The donkey has a reputation for being stubborn and unwilling. This is often because the donkey shows reluctance without displaying the body language of the horse or pony. The actual cause of the behaviour is more likely to be fear, pain, lack of motivation or clarity of instruction rather than stubbornness.

⚠ **ALERT**

The 'stubborn' donkey is more likely to be avoiding a fearful situation or lacking motivation.

RESTRAINT TECHNIQUES FOR PROCEDURES AND TREATMENT

There are several restraint techniques that are appropriate for the donkey.

Taking care to minimise stress will make restraint easier and safer for all concerned:

- Owners should be advised to bring two bonded animals together into the yard, stable or veterinary hospital because isolation from companions can cause significant stress.

- If the patient is not one of a bonded pair, there should be another calm donkey in close proximity to the patient.

- If the animal has travelled for a period of time to reach the clinic it is important to make food and water available prior to further handling.

- Both animals should be restrained with a head collar in an enclosed, quiet and safe environment.

- The use of an appropriate and well fitting head collar is essential.

Consider the use of personal protective equipment and clothing. Remember that donkeys may be more inclined to squash handlers against walls and solid objects.

The need for further restraint will vary according to the individual animal and situation.

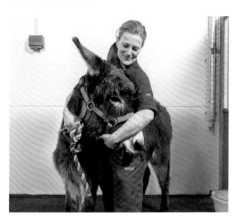 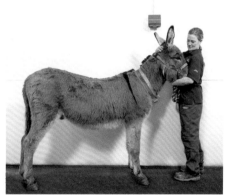

The head hold restraint is suitable for many procedures where the likely response of the donkey is known. For more unpredictable donkeys or situations, it is safer to stand to the side of the donkey in case it pushes forward.

For the head hold restraint:

- Use a two-handed head hold

17

- keep the head close to the handler's chest
- keep feet pointing towards the donkey
- keep the leading leg contacting the donkey's chest if possible
- ensure that no fingers are trapped
- ensure that the nostrils aren't occluded.

If the head hold restraint is not sufficient to carry out the procedure safely, consider:

- Sedation may be necessary.

➡ *See Chapter 16: Sedation, Anaesthesia and Analgesia for more information.*

- Distraction with a food reward during the procedure.
- Raising the head of the donkey to reduce the risk of moving forwards.
- Lifting the forelimb to limit movement.

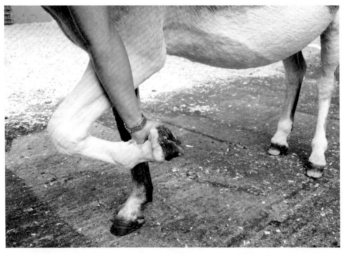

Correct leg lift to limit movement during short procedures.

- Holding a fold of skin on the neck.

⚠ **ALERT**

Ear twitching is not recommended; it is painful and can result in a fear response.

Grasping the ear, and particularly twisting the ear with a hand or rope ('ear twitching'), is not recommended. As well as being painful and potentially damaging it will lead to dangerous fear responses in the future whenever the head is approached.

Holding the nose with hands, rope or other devices ('nose twitching') has a very variable response in donkeys and is not recommended.

Moving the 'frozen' donkey

Untrained or fearful donkeys may 'freeze' or pull away from pressure. Donkeys can be trained to lead successfully using appropriate reinforcement of the desired behaviour. However, the following management strategies may be used:

- Make the environment inviting for the donkey, for example by removing objects the donkey fears, turning on lights in dark areas, opening up doorways as wide as possible, or spreading straw or other bedding material.

- Position the patient's companion at a distance and encourage the donkey to move towards its friend or walk the companion up alongside the patient.

- Use food incentives.

- Backing the donkey through doorways and into stocks, can be effective.

- Blindfolding may be appropriate but this carries the risk of inducing panic.

- A broad webbing strap behind the donkey's hindquarters can be used to prevent backwards movement and encourage forward steps.

COMMON BEHAVIOURAL PROBLEMS

> ⚠ **ALERT**
>
> 'Problem' behaviours are commonly normal behavioural responses that serve a purpose for the individual animal, but may be undesirable for the owner.

An understanding of learning theory can help improve behavioural compliance.

When behaviour cannot be easily modified it is advisable to seek the guidance of a trained professional such as a board-certified Veterinary Behaviourist or a Clinical Animal Behaviour Counsellor.

➡ *See online at* **thedonkeysanctuary.org.uk/for-professionals** *for more information on behaviour and treatment.*

Wood chewing

This is often a normal behaviour, linked to the donkey's natural browsing habit. Donkeys should have constant access to fibrous forage to fulfil their need to graze for 14—18 hours a day. Examples include straw, hay, and the bark, branches and leaves of non-poisonous plants. Slow feeders, small-holed hay nets and track systems should also be considered.

Attacking other livestock or companion animals

This can be an expression of the donkey's natural behaviour in warding off potential predators and donkeys are used as guard animals to protect livestock.

Ideally donkeys should not be housed in mixed species groups. If such housing is unavoidable, the animals should be introduced to each other gradually. It is important that all the animals have an escape route out of the field/shelter.

Difficulty handling feet

Due to their small size and narrow stature, care should be taken to hold feet as low as possible and not abducted from the body to prevent unbalancing the donkey.

Appropriate shaping plans will be needed when problems persist with foot handling.

🐴 MULES AND HINNIES

- Mules tend to have the behavioural repertoire of both horses and donkeys, if they are handled from an early age they can be very rewarding and make excellent riding and draft animals.

- Where they are not handled or trained, they initially show subtle behavioural signs of fear like the donkey, and then rapidly switch between the flight responses of a horse and the fight responses of a donkey. When the initial signs of fear are missed, these behaviours can appear explosive and violent.

- Mules can jump from a standstill.

- Due to their explosive fear responses, unhandled or stressed mules can pose a high risk to the handler.

- Mules can be trained using systematic desensitisation and counter-conditioning. In the long term this can reduce the stress for the mule and significantly improve safety for the handlers.

- It may be appropriate to slow down and take the time required to work at a pace that does not induce the panic or defence response. If physical restraint is required, ensure it is safe for all concerned and applied for as short a time as necessary.

- If the mule has not had any formal training, has previously shown any dangerous behaviour, or is stressed, the clinician should consider sedation.

- Early administration of sedatives is advised to minimise catecholamine release and improve sedation.

- Oral or IM administration of sedatives may be appropriate.

- Nose twitches can be effective for mules. However, there is much debate over their possible negative effects. For this reason, their use should be carefully considered and limited to a short length of time, for example to enable sedative administration.

- Chutes and stocks that are designed for mules are available.

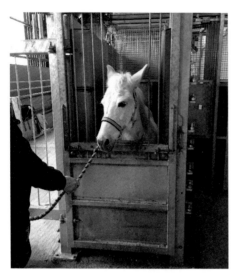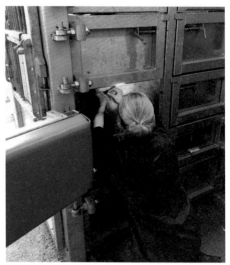

Purpose built padded stocks can be useful when handling feral mules. Multiple 'windows' allow access to different parts of the body.

ℹ️ FURTHER INFORMATION

Factsheets, research and detailed information can be found online at:
thedonkeysanctuary.org.uk/for-professionals

Burden, F. and Thiemann, A. (2015) Donkeys Are Different. *Journal of Equine Veterinary Science*, 35: 376—382.

Osthaus, B., Proops, L., Hocking, I., Burden, F. (2013) Spatial cognition and perseveration by horses, donkeys and mules in a simple A-not-B detour task. *Animal Cognition*, 16 (2): 301—305.

Murray, L.M.A. et al (2012) Pair-bonding and companion recognition in domestic donkeys, *Equus asinus. Appl. Anim. Behav. Sci.*, 143 (1): 67—74.

Proops, L., Burden, F. and Osthaus, B. (2009) Mule cognition: a case of hybrid vigour? *Animal Cognition*, 12 (1): 75—84.

Proops, L., Burden, F. and Osthaus, B. (2012) Social relations in a mixed group of mules, ponies and donkeys reflect differences in equid type. *Behavioural Processes*, 90 (3): 337—342.

Ali, A.B.A., Matoock, M.Y., Fouad, A.A. and Heleski, C.R. (2015) Are mules or donkeys better adapted for Egyptian brick kiln work? (Until we can change the kilns). *Journal of Veterinary Behavior*, 10: 158—165.

Hothersall, B. and Casey, R. (2012) Undesired behaviour in horses: A review of their development, prevention, management and association with welfare. *Equine Veterinary Education*, 24 (9): 479—485.

McGreevy, P. (2012) Equine Behaviour. A guide for Veterinarians and Equine Scientists. Saunders.

2. THE HEAD AND ORAL CAVITY

Dental disease is recorded as being the second most common clinical problem encountered in the donkey, after disorders of the feet. It has the potential to cause significant pain, which may go unrecognised in these stoic animals. Prophylactic dentistry is essential.

Note that this chapter uses the TRIADAN nomenclature and refers to a complete dental formula of 44 teeth (11 teeth in each one of the 4 quadrants): 3 incisors, 1 canine, 4 premolars (including wolf tooth) and 3 molars. The cheek teeth (CT) refer to 3 premolars and 3 molars (TRIADAN nomenclature 06 to 11).

CLINICAL EXAMINATION

ORAL AND DENTAL DISORDERS

TREATMENT

PREVENTION AND QUALITY OF LIFE

KEY POINTS

- Significant dental disease may be present in donkeys that are in good condition and show no clinical symptoms.

- A thorough visual and digital oral examination is an essential part of the clinical examination of any sick donkey.

- Excessive salivation, oral malodour, inappetence/anorexia, impaction related colic, hyperlipaemia, and weight/condition loss are often indications of a dental condition.

PREVENTION

- Regular prophylactic dental care is not always in place for the donkey but it can reduce the likelihood of significant dental disease in later years.

The digestive system of the donkey is primarily designed to obtain energy from a highly fibrous forage diet, consumed steadily throughout the day. A series of anatomical features in the head and oral cavity are directly related with the need to feed on abrasive foodstuffs.

Some of the important anatomical differences between the head and oral cavity of the donkey and those of horses and ponies are:

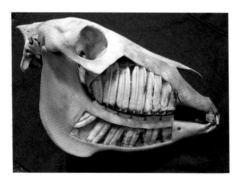

A young donkey skull demonstrating a high-crowned molarised CT, the close relationship between maxillary CT (8—11s) and nasal sinus, and the correct position of the CT, including the different angulation patterns, maintaining tight apposition of all CT at the occlusal surface. Note the presence of the curve of Spee.

- The curvature of the combined occlusal surfaces of the cheek teeth (CT), which is known as the curve of Spee, is prominent in some donkeys. In these cases teeth should not be modified in an attempt to correct the condition. They should be maintained following the jaw lines and allowing for normal, uniform clinical crown height.

- Donkeys present a greater degree of anisognathia – ie the maxilla is approximately 30% wider than the mandible (5—7% wider than in horses) at its widest point. The disproportion of width appears to stem from a narrower straight mandible rather than a wider maxilla. This greater degree of anisognathia may be related to the need to have a wider lateral excursion movement, to allow effective chewing of a diet of very rough forage. This anatomical difference is important to consider when deciding whether enamel 'overgrowths' are physiological or pathological structures in donkeys.

- In the donkey the rostral and caudal maxillary sinuses may communicate freely because they are incompletely divided by a ventrally located low bony ridge which does not extend dorsally enough to divide both sinuses.

- Donkeys have a different anatomical location for the opening of the distal nasolacrimal duct. It is small and found variably on the dorsolateral aspect of the nares, often close to the junction with the false nares. This position is potentially useful to avoid blockage with sand or dust in the habitat that the donkey evolved in.

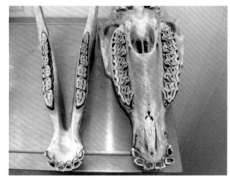

Mandible and maxilla of a donkey, where the anisognathia is evident. Note the significant differences in morphology between maxillary and mandibular CT, with maxillary CT presenting a greater surface area and containing more enamel in the form of mesial and distal infundibula.

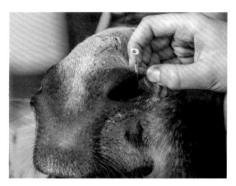

Anatomical location of the nasolacrimal duct foramen in donkeys.

CLINICAL EXAMINATION

- 0—5 years: This is the most dynamic period, with the eruption of deciduous and definitive teeth and the dental exchange process. It is advisable to carry out more frequent prophylactic examinations (every six months).

Exchange of deciduous for permanent teeth in donkeys:

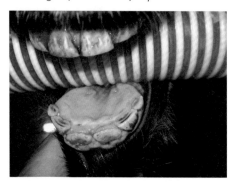 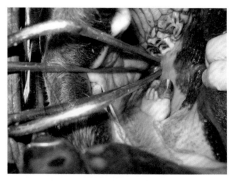

Definitive 301 and 401, erupting but not yet in contact with opposite incisors.

806 still present, but a clear demarcation between deciduous and definitive CT is evident at the gum level.

> ⚠ **ALERT**
>
> Donkeys tend to exchange the decididuous teeth 2 to 6 months later than is recorded in horses, so extra care must be taken when deciding to remove retained caps.

- 5—20 years: An annual prophylactic examination may be sufficient during this period, unless developmental problems are identified.

- 15—20 years and above: Teeth may start to suffer anatomical changes and dental disease may be secondary to other conditions. Identified dental conditions need continuous treatment and it is advisable to carry out frequent prophylactic examinations (at least every six months).

Observation

Observation is an important part of any clinical investigation and, whenever possible, donkeys should be observed in their normal environment, eating their normal diet. However, a number of donkeys will be presented at mobile clinics and this observation is not possible.

Check:

- Feeding behaviour: check the chewing movement and identify any abnormal sound or abnormal chewing pattern which may indicate restriction of free jaw excursion. This is very important to consider alongside clinical signs such as quidding or drooling.

- Feeders and drinkers: look for signs of vices or remnants of poorly chewed food, etc. Drinkers are a valuable check, because donkeys suffering from dental disorders may drop food in the drinkers while drinking, or may deliberately put forage in the water as a way to soften the food.

- Manure: look for undigested grain or, more commonly, increased fibre length.

Extraoral examination

The extraoral examination is performed as in horses and ponies, but it is important to remember that donkeys are less likely to demonstrate pain. Manual nociceptive tests (pressure tests) will result in severe and/or acute pain where disorders are present and may enable better identification and assessment of pain in this stoic animal.

Tests include:

- **Cheek pressure** is exerted bilaterally and simultaneously on the cheeks at the level of the maxillary CT by pressing the cheek against the entire CT row, starting from the level of the medial canthus of the eye and progressing rostral over the masseter muscle to the level of the nasal notch. Signs of discomfort (tossing the head) may be the result of pain from sharp CT enamel overgrowths or any other abnormal wear patterns on the vestibular/rostral aspect of the upper CT (eg displaced teeth and focal overgrowths).

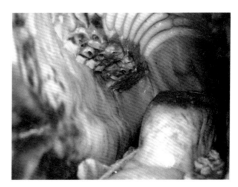

The tongue is pushed laterally toward/ against the 3rd arcade, and the right cheek pushed medially against the first arcade, simulating the nociceptive test. Note the close contact between CT and soft tissues and the presence of an ulcer at the level of 110, which may cause a violent pain response.

- **Tongue/hyoid pressure** is exerted bilaterally on the intermandibular space, pushing the body of tongue dorsally, leading to close contact between the mandibular CT and the lateral aspect of the tongue. Signs of discomfort may be the result of dental trauma at the back of the mouth causing ulcers or lacerations of the tongue, sharp CT enamel overgrowths, or lingually displaced CT.

A positive response to this test will indicate the need for conservative reduction of any enamel points. It must also lead to consideration of methods to be used for the intraoral examination; a fully opened mouth with a speculum in place will push the cheeks tightly against the CT. This will cause discomfort and may lead to soft tissue damage in extreme cases.

- **Temporomandibular joint pressure** or rostrocaudal and lateral manipulation of the mandible may result in a positive response indicating the presence of disease affecting the temporomandibular joint or more chronic and severe oral disorders.

> ⚠ **ALERT**
>
> The period of time that the mouth of the donkey is kept open during the intraoral examination and treatment must be limited in all cases, but particular care must be taken where there is any response to temporomandibular joint pressure.

Intraoral examination

The animal's general behaviour should be assessed, and a decision made on the need for sedation before completing the intraoral examination.

The intraoral examination is undertaken as in horses and ponies, and care must be taken to limit periods of time that the mouth is kept open for examination or for treatment.

It is important to flush the oral cavity using a dosing syringe before using the gag.

Unsedated donkeys may object to oral rinsing and reactions may be violent: the presence of water under pressure in the oral cavity stimulates the soft palate to contract, causing a rostral displacement of the palatopharyngeal arch, leading to a blockage of the entrance to the trachea. Animals will calm down and start breathing normally within 10 seconds, but it may be necessary to stimulate the throat region so that the donkey will swallow and relax the adjacent structures. Therefore the mouth should not be flushed with the gag on and the mouth open.

> ⚠ **ALERT**
>
> Unsedated donkeys may react violently to oral rinsing.

Many donkeys allow the intraoral examination and non-painful procedures during treatment without the need to be sedated. When working with unsedated donkeys, keeping the head high may reduce their attempts to push forward. Unsedated animals should never be left unattended with a gag in place.

Sedation, if appropriate, should be carried out as in horses and ponies, using the standard doses as stated for equines, but with more frequent top-ups.

→ *See Chapter 16: Sedation, Anaesthesia and Analgesia for more information.*

⚠ **ALERT**

Regular-size donkeys may be treated with standard equine dental equipment. Miniature donkeys may require specialized, smaller-size tools.

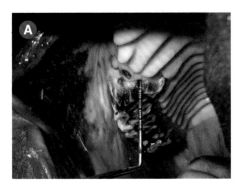 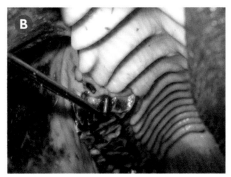

Use of dental probe (A) to assess the depth of a diastema with periodontal pocket (B) in a case of a supernumerary 106. The measurement of these pockets is mandatory to correctly evaluate the degree of attachment loss in cases of periodontal disease. Supernumerary teeth are usually maxillary distomolars, but may occur in other places.

⚠ **ALERT**

Always be aware of the possibility of infection with rabies. Dumb rabies can cause hypersalivation in the donkey. Take precautions when carrying out an oral examination.

Some important points to note for the examination of a donkey are:

- In donkeys with absent or a few stable incisors, it may be preferable to use ground-out incisor plates rather than traditional 'gum' bars, to avoid trauma to the interdental space, which may occur even when they are padded.

- It is suggested that ventral curvature of the incisors is a normal feature in donkeys. However, studies suggest it is an acquired disorder, increasing significantly with age and possibly due to disorders in the CT that affect the normal movement of the jaw. If indicated, phased correction is advised, restoring normal incisor conformation, but care must be taken to avoid loss of incisor occlusion.

- In donkeys it is normal to find up to 4 wolf teeth (one per arcade). These teeth should not contact or interfere with a correctly used bit.

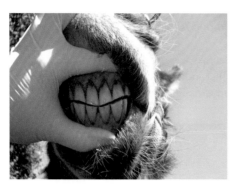

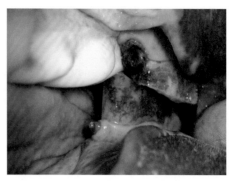

Acquired ventral curvature in the occlusal surface of incisors in an adult donkey, as a consequence of other concomitant disorders in the CT, affecting the normal movement of the jaw.

Presence of maxillary and mandibular wolf teeth in a donkey. The presence of wolf teeth in donkeys is common, particularly the upper ones. When present, the mandibular wolf teeth are usually smaller. Note the presence of a peripheral caries affecting 205.

Ancillary diagnostic tests

These tests are similar to those used in horses and ponies, with radiography being the most commonly used diagnostic method. Rhinoscopy may be useful but it is important to remember that the nasal passages of the donkey are smaller than similar sized horses and ponies, so good lubrication and the correct diameter endoscope is important.

ORAL AND DENTAL DISORDERS

There is limited robust published information on donkey oral health and dental disease. However, those studies that are available indicate that a wide range of pathology is seen in a significant proportion of animals in all the environments in which they are kept. The pathology often increases in incidence and severity with age and may be more prevalent in certain populations or breeds. Individual animals often present with multiple disorders.

➔ *See online at **thedonkeysanctuary.org.uk/for-professionals** for a list of definitions of the most common dental disorders in donkeys.*

Developmental disorders of the teeth

Developmental disorders of teeth in donkeys are similar to those found in horses and ponies.

Those disorders with donkey specific differences include:

Craniofacial abnormalities which need early detection and treatment to prevent development into more severe conditions. These may have a genetic basis and breeding from affected animals is not recommended.

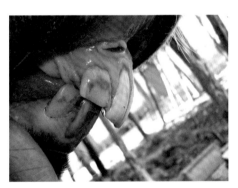 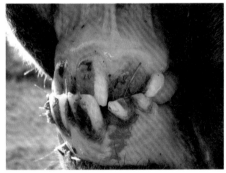

Extreme cases of overbite and underbite in donkeys. In these cases of craniofacial abnormalities there is a clear mechanical blockage interfering with the correct chewing movement. Note the presence of a retained 702. The lack of contact with the ipsilateral opposite tooth in these cases may favour the occurrence of retentions.

Dental dysplasia is relatively uncommon.

Polyodontia is relatively uncommon but very important. Fully erupted supernumerary teeth are reported with an increasing prevalence in elderly donkeys. This suggests a late-onset eruption process. Supernumerary teeth are commonly located in the caudal aspects of the maxillary CT in the donkey and are therefore easily missed.

Retained deciduous teeth will mainly affect the donkey between 2.5 and 5 years of age. A knowledge of eruption times of the teeth for donkeys is important to avoid premature removal of deciduous teeth, which may affect the underlying developing permanent tooth. Recent studies show that teeth fragments are more commonly found on the medial aspect of the CT rows in donkeys, so extra care is needed during the extraction of these fragments to avoid laceration of the great palatine artery. The most common deciduous teeth to be retained are central incisors (01s) and deciduous 08s.

Eruption cysts are relatively common.

Abnormal dental eruption, displacements and developmental diastemata are all found in donkeys. A high prevalence of 03s distally displaced has been described. These abnormalities can increase the likelihood of complicated fractures in the displaced teeth and food entrapment, with associated gingivitis and periodontitis.

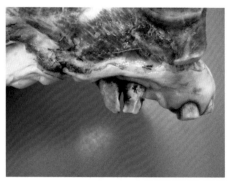

Post-mortem examination finding of a double 104 in a donkey.

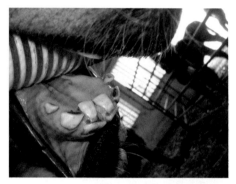

Retained central mandibular incisors (701 and 801), displaced lingually as a result of the eruption of the definitive 301 and 401. Note the presence of open diastemata affecting all deciduous mandibular incisors, probably due to lack of rostro-mesial compression. This clinical situation may increase the chance of dental fractures.

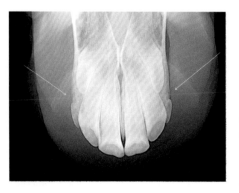

Radiographic image of the maxillary incisors, highlighting the anatomical position of the incisors ('hand fan' shape), promoting the rostro-mesial compression and maintaining the ability of the incisor arcade to act as a single unit, avoiding the formation of developmental diastemata.

Acquired disorders of the teeth

Those disorders with donkey specific differences include:

Hypodontia (loss of teeth) is seen in both incisors and CT and is common in donkeys and particularly in the geriatric. This may be due to periodontal disease.

Abnormalities of wear increase with age and affect the occlusal surface of both incisors and CT. It is the most common disorder of CT; mainly seen as enamel overgrowths affecting all CT.

Ventral curvature which is an age-related acquired disorder. Studies report a 10% prevalence in donkeys less than 10 years old and up to 80% in animals older than 25 years. It is probably secondary to CT disorders interfering with the correct chewing movement. Phased correction is advised, balancing and correcting the disorders of CT, while restoring the occlusal normal incisor conformation.

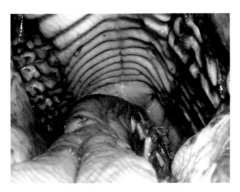

An extreme case of shear mouth, affecting the left arcades of a donkey. Note the asymmetric aspect of the hard palate, indicating alterations in the palatine bone. Also note the soft tissue trauma in the palatine mucosa, caused by the close contact with the mandibular CT. Treatment must focus on conservative elimination of the sharp abnormal structures in the affected arcades, avoiding soft tissue trauma, and keeping the unaffected arcades balanced.

Focal overgrowths affecting the 06s and the 11s; mainly found in those donkeys with some degree of incisor malocclusion.

Overgrowth of the complete tooth due to poor or absent occlusal contact is not uncommon and frequently bilateral. These overgrown teeth interfere with normal chewing movement and may predispose to the development of **wave mouth** or **shear mouth**.

Studies in working equids suggest a high prevalence of CT enamel overgrowth and the majority of associated soft tissue lesions are located on the cheeks beside the maxillary 06s and 07s. This corresponds with areas where halters may exert pressure and may indicate a different aetiology for this disorder. It may be that higher protruding enamel on the CT is physiological and a normal feature for donkeys, in which case the pain response to the nociceptive tests (cheek and tongue/hyoid pressure) may be used as an indicator for the need for correction of enamel overgrowths.

Early detection and treatment of abnormalities of wear can avoid its development into more severe conditions.

Dental displacements are recorded. Molar displacements, with diastemata formation and the potential for soft tissue trauma are seen and O6 CT is the most commonly affected. If not treated, these displacements may be severe and, if periodontal disease is not advanced, these teeth may have very solid attachments.

Diastemata with food entrapment and associated periodontal disease are a very painful disorder. Acquired diastemata are a common disorder of the donkey, affecting mainly mandibular CT. They are an age related disorder, increasing in extent and prevalence with age.

A thorough visual and digital oral examination is essential to investigate clinical signs such as; excessive salivation, oral malodour, inappetence/anorexia, colic (especially impaction), hyperlipaemia, and weight/condition loss.

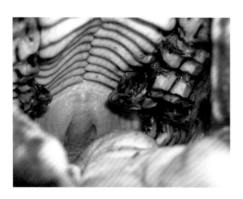

Palatal displacement affecting 109 and 209, with 210 and 211 displaced buccally. Note the diastemata formation affecting all interproximal spaces between 208 and 211, with food entrapment and periodontal disease. 211 also presents overgrowth of the complete tooth.

Periodontal disease (PD) is a common disorder, as in horses and ponies.

Periodontal disease in donkey cheek teeth demonstrates an age related increase in severity, simultaneous to an higher number of affected teeth compared to horses.

Periodontal disease in donkey incisor teeth demonstrates no age related increase in severity, but an increase in the number of incisors affected.

Calculus was recorded as the main predisposing factor for incisor PD. It may be reversible if the calculus is removed at an early stage.

More severe cases can lead to attachment loss and periodontitis.

Diastemata and retained deciduous incisors are related to PD in the definitive incisors. In CT almost 90% of teeth diagnosed with PD were caused by diastemata.

Other less common causes of PD include peripheral caries, damage in the normal tight junction between gingiva and peripheral cementum at the gingival margin, leading to attachment loss in some cases, and retained deciduous CT.

Caries may affect all dental components at a peripheral and infundibular level. This disorder has been shown to increase with age. Prevalence and severity of the degree observed, and cause, are similar to those seen in horses and ponies.

Calculus is often related to the presence of other dental conditions as in horses and ponies. Elderly donkeys may present with considerable malodorous deposits at the canines and incisors, but also around the maxillary premolars adjacent to the ostium of the parotid duct.

There appears to be less sexual dimorphism relating to the canines than demonstrated in horses and ponies, and both male and female donkeys may be affected.

Fractures are reported to have a variable prevalence, with the higher prevalence possibly related to biting hard objects during daily grazing on poor and stony soils. The majority of fractures in incisors were uncomplicated, affecting only the external components of the teeth.

Due to the anatomy of CT, all fractures (even small slab fractures) have pulpar exposure (ie are complicated fractures), so careful clinical inspection of these areas is important, using dental probes and a mirror.

In one study some donkeys were observed with small fractures in the rostral aspect of 06s that appeared to be the site of former small focal overgrowths that fractured under the high pressures of normal equine mastication. The pulp horn inevitably involved appeared to be sealed off.

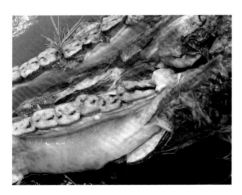

Complicated idiopathic dental fracture affecting 311 found in a post-mortem examination. This almost sagittal fracture resulted in bacterial invasion of the pulp and apical infection. Also note the presence of several diastemata with food entrapment and CT displacements.

Apical infection presents in donkeys as in horses and ponies.

Soft tissues lesions

Lesions may be seen in the soft tissues and are common in working donkeys. Inappropriate and poorly fitting bits or restraint systems with tight nosebands are some examples where soft tissues can be compressed against the teeth, causing lesions.

➡ *See online at* **thedonkeysanctuary.org.uk/ for-professionals** *for more information in The Good Harness Guide.*

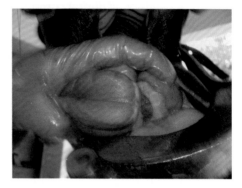

Severe laceration affecting the tongue of a mule, caused by the incorrect use of a traditional bit in Morocco.

TREATMENT

Treatment follows established best practice in horses and ponies.

A treatment plan is essential when treating significant dental disease. The plan should consider staging procedures in order to avoid post-treatment stress, anorexia and potential hyperlipaemia.

⚠ **ALERT**

> Where possible avoid multiple extractions in one session. The sudden reduced function, in addition to possible stress and pain, may cause acute inappetence.

A full clinical examination, preferably including haematology and biochemistry screens, is strongly recommended to inform a treatment plan, particularly in elderly or sick donkeys or those with potentially reduced appetite.

It is preferable to perform staged reductions over time rather than one corrective procedure in all but the most minor overgrowths.

⚠ **ALERT**

> Drastic reduction may result in exposure of pulp and irreversible dental pain.

Care must be taken to avoid direct or indirect pulp exposure during dental reductions. Whilst working on the occlusal surfaces; the staining of the secondary dentine may lighten in colour but must remain visible at all regions of the crown.

As donkeys typically live longer than horses, it is possible to perform minor reductions and regain occlusion in animals in their late teens/early twenties. It is, however, occasionally best for the elderly patient to allow minor focal overgrowths to remain in order to allow as much occlusion as possible.

It is not uncommon in elderly donkeys, particularly on the maxillary arcades, that once one tooth is extracted, two or three others lose their stability and also require extraction. Radiographs may be helpful to identify such cases prior to treatment.

Appropriate analgesia should be considered and prescribed.

➡ *See Chapter 17: Pharmacology and Therapeutics for more information.*

Donkeys with dental disease or undergoing dental treatment will frequently require dietary modification.

➡ *See Chapter 18: Nutrition for more information.*

PREVENTION AND QUALITY OF LIFE

Dentistry should be prophylactic. A regular programme of routine examinations and care will allow the early diagnosis and treatment of oral and dental disorders and avoid their development into potentially significant pathology.

- Good dental care has proven benefits for the health and welfare of donkeys.

- All donkeys require a regular dental care programme that includes full oral examination, appropriately adapted to the individual and its age.

- A full clinical examination and assessment should be undertaken before treating significant dental disorders, particularly in elderly donkeys.

- Dental disease is an integral component of any quality of life assessment.

- Diets should be modified appropriately to avoid problems of colic, choke (oesophageal obstruction) and weight loss.

Consideration must be given to the quality of life of the donkey when considering any treatment plan. Important questions are:

- What is the overall aim of treatment and what procedures are required?

- Can they be competently undertaken with or without hospitalisation?

- What is the likely recovery period and what will post-procedural function be?

- How will pain and diet be managed?

- What other issues does the donkey present with?

Many clinical situations may have a direct impact on the quality of life of donkeys, with some being life threatening, as described for cases of extreme craniofacial abnormalities in new-born donkeys.

In older animals, CT loss, dental functional capacity and average faecal fibre length provides useful information for the quality of life assessment, treatment planning, and post-procedural care/management considerations, in addition to dealing with owner expectations.

The location of missing CT and the presence of multiple adjacent tooth loss has a bearing on longevity.

🐴 MULES AND HINNIES

The temperament of mules may make intraoral examination difficult without sedation. Mules may require different doses for effective sedation.

The anatomical location of the nasolacrimal duct is very variable in the mule.

ℹ FURTHER INFORMATION

Factsheets, research and detailed information can be found online at:
thedonkeysanctuary.org.uk/for-professionals, including a full list of short
definitions of the most common dental disorders affecting donkeys.

du Toit, N., Burden, F.A. and Dixon, P.M. (2009) Clinical dental examinations of
357 donkeys in the UK. Part 1: Prevalence of dental disorders. *Equine Vet. J.*
41(4). 390—394.

du Toit, N., Burden, F.A. and Dixon, P.M. (2009) Clinical dental examinations
of 357 donkeys in the UK. Part 2: Epidemiological studies on the potential
relationships between different dental disorders, and between dental disease
and systemic disorders. *Equine Vet. J.* 41(4). 395—400.

du Toit, N., Burden, F.A. and Dixon, P.M. (2008) Clinical dental findings in 203
working donkeys in Mexico. *Vet J.* 178(3). 380—386.

du Toit, N. and Dixon, P.M. (2012) Common dental disorders in the donkey.
Equine Vet. Educ. 24(1). 45—51.

du Toit, N., Gallagher, J., Burden, F.A. and Dixon, P.M. (2008) *Post mortem* survey
of dental disorders in 349 donkeys from an aged population (2005—2006).
Part 1: Prevalence of specific dental disorders. *Equine Vet. J.* 40(3). 204—208.

du Toit, N., Gallagher, J., Burden, F.A. and Dixon, P.M. (2008) *Post mortem* survey
of dental disorders in 349 donkeys from an aged population (2005-2006). Part
2: Epidemiological studies. *Equine Vet. J.* 40(3). 209—213.

du Toit, N., Kempson, S.A. and Dixon, P.M. (2008) Donkey dental anatomy.
Part 1: Gross and computed axial tomography examinations. *Vet J.* 176 (3).
338—344.

Morrow, L.D., Smith, K.C., Piercy, R.J., du Toit, N., Burden, F.A., Olmos, G.,
Gregory, N.G. and Verheyen, K.L.P. (2010) Retrospective analysis of *post mortem*
findings in 1,444 aged donkeys. *J. Comp. Pathol.* 144 (2-3). 145—156.

Rodrigues, J.B., Araújo, S., Sanroman-Llorens, F., Bastos, E., San Roman, F. and
Viegas, C. (2013) A clinical survey evaluating the prevalence of incisor disorders
in Zamorano-Leonés and Mirandês donkeys (*Equus asinus*). *J Equine Vet. Sci.* 33
(9). 710—718.

Rodrigues, J.B., Dixon, P.M., Bastos, E., San Roman, F. and Viegas, C. (2013) A
clinical survey on the prevalence and types of cheek teeth disorders present
in 400 Zamorano-Leonés and 400 Mirandês donkeys (*Equus asinus*). *Vet. Rec.*
173(23). 581—588.

Rodrigues, J.B., Ferreira, L.M., Bastos, E., San Roman, F., Viegas, C.A. and Santos,
A.S. (2013) Influence of dental correction on nociceptive test responses, faecal
appearance, body condition score and apparent digestibility coefficient for dry matter
of Zamorano-Leonés donkeys (*Equus asinus*). *J. Anim. Sci.* 91(10). 4765—4771.

Rodrigues, J.B., Sanroman-Llorens, F., Bastos, E., San Roman, F. and Viegas, C.
(2013) Polyodontia in donkeys. *Equine Vet. Educ.* 25(7): 363—367.

3. THE GASTROINTESTINAL SYSTEM

Most conditions of the gastrointestinal system present as in horses and ponies.

The prevalence of colic varies according to the donkey population and can be a cause of significant mortality.

There is a high risk of hyperlipaemia and gastric ulceration secondary to periods of inappetence or starvation.

By recognising the importance of subtle behavioural clues and a thorough diagnostic evaluation, donkeys with colic may be treated effectively. Treatment of secondary hyperlipaemia and gastric ulceration will ensure that the donkey has an improved chance of making a full recovery. Key preventative health measures will reduce the incidence of colic.

Surgical treatment of colic is not covered in this chapter, because the approach is the same as for the horse and pony.

CLINICAL EXAMINATION

DIAGNOSTIC PROCEDURES

COMMON CONDITIONS

PREVENTION

KEY POINTS

- Detecting colic can be difficult and/or delayed in donkeys due to their stoic nature and the subtle clinical signs displayed.

- Secondary hyperlipaemia is always a risk with colic/inappetence.

- A rectal examination is strongly advised when this can be safely undertaken.

- Obesity can complicate taking a peritoneal tap, obtaining a good ultrasound image, and surgical access to the abdomen.

- There is a strong association between dental disease and colic.

PREVENTION

- Good preventative management practices will reduce the incidence of colic, particularly regular dental care, appropriate diet, and strategic parasite control.

The gastrointestinal system of the donkey is similar in anatomy to that of horses and ponies.

The risk factors for the occurrence of colic in the donkey depend on the population under investigation.

Working donkeys globally are more likely to have an inadequate water supply, dry or inappropriate feeding practices, and poor parasite control strategies, all of which will increase the risk of colic.

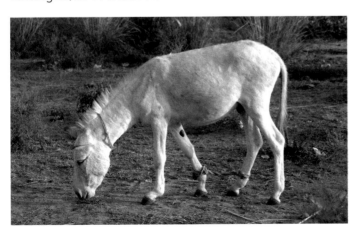

A working donkey – scavenging on inappropriate feed from rubbish dumped in the area.

Companion donkeys may not receive good preventative treatment such as regular dental examinations and effective parasite control strategies. This will increase the risk of colic, as will inappropriate changes in diet and management.

In the UK studies have shown that the most common type of colic encountered in the donkey is impaction colic of the pelvic flexure and caecum.

The common risk factors for impaction colic included:

- increasing age
- dental disease
- access to concentrate feed
- reduced water intake.

CLINICAL EXAMINATION

➔ *See Appendix 1 for a summary of the clinical examination.*

A thorough clinical examination of the donkey must always include a period of observation of their behaviour. Due to the often delayed recognition and subtle signs of a sick donkey the animal may be more compromised than expected or than it initially appears. It is important to watch how the donkey responds to a feed, and whether it eats and drinks effectively.

The history will help to identify any risk factors and changes that would predispose the donkey to colic. Any preventative management such as worming or dental examinations should be noted.

> ⚠ **ALERT**
>
> **Inappetence or anorexia may result in hyperlipaemia. This can complicate the clinical picture and make diagnosis of colic challenging.**

Donkeys can be challenging patients to treat when they present with colic because the nature of the donkey's pain-related behaviours will often mask clinical signs and the subtle changes in behaviour rarely give an indication of the urgency of the condition. Inappetence or anorexia will quickly induce hyperlipaemia. This complicates the donkey's behavioural and physiological responses and makes diagnosis and treatment more difficult.

➔ *See Chapter 7: Hyperlipaemia and the Endocrine System for more information.*

Remember that the physiological parameters of the donkey differ from those of horses and ponies.

> ℹ **INFORMATION**
>
> **Adult donkey physiological parameters**
> - **Temperature:** 36.5—37.8°C
> - **Pulse:** 36—52 beats/minute
> - **Respiration:** normally 20 breaths/minute but with a range of 12—28 breaths/minute

A pulse rate of over 70 would indicate severe disease, hypovolaemic shock or pain.

Donkeys are reported to have an increased ability to tolerate dehydration; capillary refill time and pulse quality may remain more normal than expected in the face of fluid loss.

Clinical and behavioural signs

The behaviour of donkeys in response to pain is different to that of horses and ponies, with the donkey often showing more subtle behavioural indicators of pain in response to equivalent pain stimuli.

➔ *See Chapter 1: Behaviour for more information.*

Typical colic signs in the donkey include:

- dullness

- isolation from companion or group

- reduced appetite and ineffective eating

- recumbency.

Further indicators of pain include a lack of ear movement and lowered head carriage.

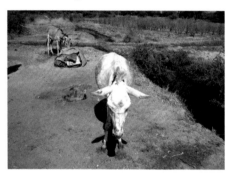

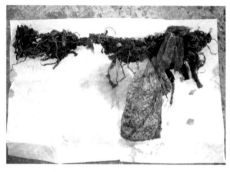

A dull donkey showing typical signs of colic, depression, low head posture and immobile ears.

The plastic rubbish recovered from the donkey.

Donkeys with severe abdominal crises may present more acutely and show rolling, sweating and groaning. In severe cases terminally ill or exhausted donkeys may be unresponsive.

The typical signs of colic in the donkey are often vague and non-specific. The clinician should rule out colic by means of a thorough clinical examination whenever a dull donkey is examined.

Issues may arise with the small size of the donkey, making clinicians wary of performing basic clinical procedures such as a rectal examination and nasogastric intubation. Obesity can impede effective ultrasonography and peritoneal taps.

There is little space in the lumbar fossa for ultrasound examination of deeper structures, and fat deposits can complicate imaging.

DIAGNOSTIC PROCEDURES

A dental examination using a Hausmann gag (oral speculum) should be performed as there is a strong association between dental disease and colic. It may not be appropriate to treat any underlying dental disorder until the colic is resolved.

Stomach tubing should be carried out using either a pony or foal stomach tube to check for reflux. The prominent large nasopharyngeal recess may make the procedure more difficult.

A rectal examination should be performed if safe to do so. Most donkeys tolerate the procedure well but some may require restraint and/or sedation. Good lubrication will aid the procedure and spasmolytic medication such as butylscopolamine can be used where appropriate to facilitate the examination.

While the clinician may be unable to palpate the abdomen extensively, useful information such as faecal consistency and mucosal hydration can be determined, even from a limited rectal examination.

An abdominal ultrasound may assist in identifying abdominal lesions in small donkeys, although subcutaneous fat may obscure detail.

A peritoneal tap can be difficult due to thick adipose deposits along the ventral body wall. This procedure may require use of a catheter, spinal needle or teat cannula in combination with ultrasonic guidance if available. The needle/trocar needs to be long enough to pass through the ventral abdominal fat, which can be up to 14cm in thickness.

A faecal sample can be used to assess endoparasite burdens and fibre length of forage. Dry faecal consistency or an excess of mucus may reflect prolonged transit time and developing hyperlipaemia.

> ⚠ **ALERT**
>
> Consider hyperlipaemia in all cases of colic, either as a primary factor leading to ileus, or as a secondary complication due to the reduction in appetite.

A serum sample to check for triglyceride levels is advisable because hyperlipaemia can be a complicating factor in all cases of colic, either as a primary factor leading to ileus, or as a secondary complication due to inappetence. If there is any doubt about the donkey's nutritional intake, it is preferable to provide energy enterally or parenterally whilst waiting for laboratory results.

A donkey should not undergo surgery for colic until the triglyceride status has been evaluated.

➜ *See Chapter 7: Hyperlipaemia and the Endocrine System for more information.*

COMMON CONDITIONS

Conditions related to upper GI tract: stomach and small intestine

Donkeys are susceptible to **gastric ulceration** and the risk is increased during periods of inappetence, hyperlipaemia and when fed intermittent concentrate feeds. Diagnosis and treatment options are similar to those for the horse and pony, with the caveat that prolonged fasting to ensure gastric emptying prior to gastroscopy can put donkeys at further risk of hyperlipaemia.

Gastric impaction or delayed gastric emptying are seen secondary to liver disease or generalised ileus, or as a primary condition in certain populations of donkeys with access to poor, dry feedstuffs or foreign bodies such as plastic bags.

Small intestinal lesions are uncommon but can be diagnosed and managed as in the horse and pony. Despite the fact that many donkeys are overweight, strangulating lipomas appear to be a rare cause of colic in the donkey.

Parascaris impactions have been found in donkeys carrying heavy burdens of this parasite.

Conditions related to lower GI tract: caecum to rectum

Impaction of the pelvic flexure and caecum are very commonly identified problems. Studies have shown that the mortality of donkeys with impaction colic is higher than that of horses and ponies. This may be due to a number of factors including delay in presentation of disease, concurrent hyperlipaemia, and concurrent medical problems in the study population affecting treatment decisions – for example, geriatric disorders.

Most donkeys with impaction colic present with only low grade signs of discomfort and a significant number will have a degree of hyperlipaemia. When treating these animals enteral feeding by stomach tube (foal or pony sized is advised) along with the use of laxatives.

An appropriate solution would be three litres of warm water with electrolytes, glucose, magnesium or sodium sulphate, and a high-fibre nutritional supplement such as a ground instant oat breakfast cereal – for example, Ready Brek. The laxative may only need to be given on one or two occasions (if more than once then it is preferable to use sodium sulphate). The nutritional support may be required for longer. Withholding all feed can exacerbate hyperlipaemia and ileus, so typically grass or soft mashes should be offered.

> ⚠️ **ALERT**
>
> With all cases of colic, the donkey undergoing treatment needs to be kept in close proximity to its bonded companion, to prevent separation stress which may exacerbate anorexia and hyperlipaemia.

Large intestine displacements and volvulus can occur in donkeys. Some animals will show obvious signs of pain, in others it may be less evident and may present later in the course of disease.

Colitis does not often present with diarrhoea. It may present with weight loss, dullness, pyrexia, tachycardia and ventral oedema due to hypoalbuminaemia. In acute severe cases signs of abdominal pain such as rolling may be seen.

The causes are the same as in horses and ponies, but cyathostomes should always be considered, especially as donkeys often have irregular, or no, parasite control.

Infectious diseases must also be ruled out, such as salmonella and clostridia, and it is important to note that diarrhoea is not always present.

Typhlocolitis is a serious medical emergency in the donkey, with generally poor outcomes despite intensive treatments.

If a primary cause can be found, then specific treatment can be initiated – for example, treatment of larval cyathostominosis. Otherwise treatment will be as for the horse and pony, with the complication of hyperlipaemia included as a poor prognostic factor.

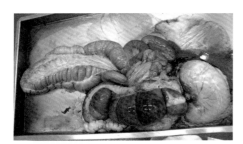 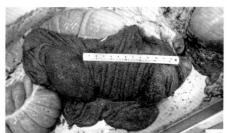

A multifocal to coalescing, severe, ulcerative and fibrinonecrotic typhlocolitis.

Colic unrelated to GI tract

As the signs of colic may be subtle, the list of differential diagnoses for a donkey with non-specific dullness is extensive.

In geriatric donkeys **abdominal neoplasia** is a significant cause of low-grade, recurrent colic, episodes. In a study of older donkeys, abdominal neoplasia involving either the gastrointestinal tract, liver, kidney or female reproductive system was found in 9.5% of donkeys examined post-mortem.

Typical cases can be hard to diagnose, especially if the donkey is on pain relief medication.

Colic symptoms have been displayed by donkeys with pyometra, enlarged ovaries and urolithiasis, underlining the importance of a rectal examination in all cases of colic.

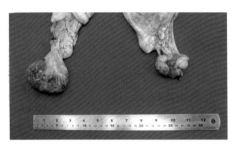 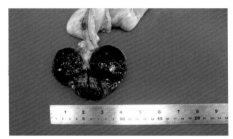

Ovarian pathology associated with low grade colic. This is an ovarian haematoma, most likely a haemorrhagic anovulatory follicle. There was also associated serosanguineous peritoneal effusion.

PREVENTION

The preventative health measures listed below have been proven to reduce the incidence of colic:

- providing regular dental checks and appropriate treatment

- feeding fibre appropriate for dental health – for example, short chop for geriatric donkeys

- supplying bedding materials appropriate for dental health (because donkeys will eat bedding)

- implementing all changes in diet and management gradually over a two week period

- providing constant trickle feed fibre and adequate exercise

- applying strategic parasite control

- providing fresh water.

🫏 **MULES AND HINNIES**

Mules appear to show an increased repertoire of pain behaviours and therefore may show more obvious signs of colic.

Mules may also be less susceptible to hyperlipaemia as a secondary complication of colic.

ℹ️ **FURTHER INFORMATION**

Factsheets, research and detailed information can be found online at: *thedonkeysanctuary.org.uk/for-professionals*

The Working Equid Veterinary Manual: *thebrooke.org/for-professionals/working-equid-veterinary-manual*

Cox R, Burden F, Proudman C, Trawford A.F, Pinchbeck. G.L (2010) Demographics, management and health of donkeys in the UK. *Veterinary Record* 166, 552-6.

du Toit N., Gallagher J., Burden F.A. and Dixon P.M. (2008) Post mortem survey of dental disorders in 349 donkeys from an aged population (2005–2006). Part 1: Prevalence of specific dental disorders. *Equine Veterinary Journal* 40, 204-208.

du Toit N., Burden F. and Dixon P.M. (2009a) Clinical dental examinations of 357 donkeys in the UK: Part 1: Prevalence of dental disorders. *Equine Veterinary Journal* 41.

du Toit N., Burden F. and Dixon, P.M. (2009b) Clinical dental examinations of 357 donkeys in the UK: Part 2: Epidemiological studies on the potential relationships between different dental disorders, and between dental disease and systemic disorders. *Equine Veterinary Journal* 41.

Burden, F.A., Gallagher, J., Thiemann, A.K. and Trawford, A.F. (2009) Necropsy survey of gastric ulcers in a population of aged donkeys: prevalence, lesion description and risk factors. *Animal* 3 (2) 287—293.

Cox, R., Burden, F., Gosden, L., Proudman, C., Trawford, A., Pinchbeck, G. (2009) Case control study to investigate risk factors for impaction colic in donkeys in the UK. *Preventative veterinary medicine* 92 179—187.

McGorum, B.C., Pirie, R.S. (2010) Asinine typhlocolitis; 'scouring' the literature for diagnostic and aetiological clues. *Equine Veterinary Education* 22 (2), 58—59.

Morrow, L.D., Smith, K.C., Piercy, R.J., du Toit, N., Burden, F.A., Olmos, G., Gregory, N.G., Verheyen, K.L.P. (2010) Retrospective analysis of post–mortem findings in 1,444 aged donkeys. *Journal of Comparative Pathology* 144 (2—3) 145—156.

Thiemann, A.K., Rickards, K., Getachew, A.M. and Paraschou, G. (2017) Colic in the donkey, Wiley publishers etc.

4. THE RESPIRATORY SYSTEM

In general, many diseases of the respiratory system in donkeys can be investigated and managed in a similar way to horses and ponies. Knowledge of donkey specific problems and anatomy can aid in the approach to diagnosis and treatment.

Respiratory disease is a significant cause of morbidity and mortality in the donkey. As the donkey does not often perform at speed and has an insensitive cough reflex it may be easy to miss early disease. It is often the case that preventative health measures, such as administering anthelmintics and vaccinations, are not applied as rigorously as in horses and ponies. Examination of such cases needs to be detailed and thorough, and treatment plans created with appreciation of donkey specific differences.

CLINICAL EXAMINATION

INFECTIOUS DISEASES

PARASITIC DISEASES

OTHER CONDITIONS OF THE UPPER RESPIRATORY TRACT

OTHER CONDITIONS OF THE LOWER RESPIRATORY TRACT

PREVENTION

KEY POINTS

- The donkey has an insensitive cough reflex and may not show many symptoms of disease.

- There is a risk of missing respiratory disease in its early stages due to the stoic nature of the donkey and especially in those which are not athletically challenged.

- There is a high risk of hyperlipaemia where pyrexia is seen with severe respiratory disease.

- Tracheal collapse, lung fibrosis and neoplasia are important differential diagnoses in the geriatric donkey.

- Donkeys have different baseline physiological parameters.

PREVENTION

Reduce the risk of disease by:

- the use of regular strategic anthelmintic and dental treatments and vaccination.

- introducing biosecurity measures including isolating and screening of new arrivals.

The donkey has evolved to live in an environment with limited resources and as a result they often form small groups, live in pairs or live solitary lives. This makes communication important and the bray is extremely loud and carries over long distances, allowing donkey groups to communicate with relatively isolated groups or pairs.

The characteristic loud bray is facilitated by a short nasopharyngeal airway which is constricted in the middle and flared dorsally and ventrally.

Some of the important anatomical variations from horses and ponies are:

- The nasopharyngeal airway is short, constricted in the middle and flared dorsally and ventrally.

- The distal nasolacrimal duct opening is small and found variably on the dorsolateral aspect of the nares, often close to the junction with the false nares. This position is potentially useful to avoid blockage with sand or dust in the habitat donkeys evolved to inhabit.

- The nasal passages are narrow.

- The nasopharyngeal recess (a diverticulum of the pharyngeal mucosa lying between the guttural pouches) is enlarged into a pouch 2—3cm across and 4—6cm long (in the horse this is 2.5cm long).

- The epiglottis is short and more pointed and the laryngeal opening tilted more caudally.

- Dark pigmentation in the larynx and upper third of the oesophagus is a normal variation.

- The paranasal sinuses are smaller and do not extend as far rostrally.

- The rostral and caudal compartment of the maxillary sinus is divided by a low, bony ridge, so the septum is incomplete.

- A small (1—1.5cm) trephine is required for accessing the frontal and caudal maxillary sinus due to the short length of the facial crest.

➔ *See Chapter 2: The Head and Oral Cavity for more information on the sinuses.*

It is also important to remember that unplanned and inbred mating is not uncommon and therefore congenital defects should be considered in certain situations.

CLINICAL EXAMINATION

The investigation for respiratory tract disease in the donkey will follow similar lines to that for horses and ponies, but it is important to consider:

- the specific anatomy of the donkey

- the different behaviours and temperaments of the donkey

- differences in the aetiology and incidence of disease related to workload and breed.

> ⚠ **ALERT**
>
> The donkey has a stoic nature and often has low demands on its stamina and performance, so it may not demonstrate the early signs typical of respiratory disease. Problems may not be detected until disease is more advanced.

➜ *See Appendix 1 for a summary of the clinical examination.*

Specific points to note when examining the donkey for respiratory disease are:

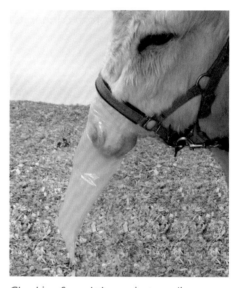

Checking for subtle respiratory disease using a re-breathing bag in a donkey.

- A full examination of the donkey should include the use of a re-breathing bag to accentuate subtle lung sounds, especially in obese donkeys where fat deposits muffle sounds.

- The donkey has an insensitive cough reflex and may not demonstrate many symptoms of disease.

- The donkey has anatomical differences which are significant to the examination for respiratory disease.

- Tracheal collapse and deformities are seen in geriatric donkeys, and tracheal auscultation and palpation are useful.

- Inspiratory and expiratory dyspnoea with absent/reduced lung sounds suggest fibrosing lung disease.

- Lungworm (*Dictyocaulus arnfieldii*) causes asymptomatic infections in the donkey, and can be diagnosed using faecal examination (Baermann technique).

Remember that secondary hyperlipaemia must be considered as a

possibility in all disease states causing stress and loss of appetite, particularly the infectious and pyrexic respiratory diseases.

Remember that the physiological parameters of the donkey differ from those of horses and ponies.

ℹ INFORMATION

Adult donkey physiological parameters

- **Temperature:** 36.5—37.8°C

- **Pulse:** 36—52 beats/minute

- **Respiration:** normally 20 breaths/minute but with a range of 12—28 breaths/minute

---

INFECTIOUS DISEASES

The donkey is susceptible to the same range of respiratory pathogens as the horse and pony.

Unlike the horse and pony, donkeys are rarely vaccinated and this failure to use a prevention programme means that there is a higher risk of infection.

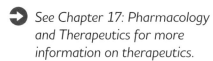 See Chapter 10: Infectious Diseases for more information.

Due to the difference in metabolism of certain drugs, treatment protocols with antibiotics and anti-inflammatories may need to be amended.

See Chapter 17: Pharmacology and Therapeutics for more information on therapeutics.

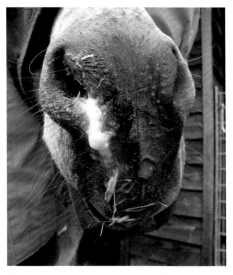

Profuse nasal discharge should be investigated promptly in the donkey to rule out infectious disease.

Equine Influenza presents with the same clinical signs as seen in horses and ponies, however there are reports that donkeys may be more severely affected.

⚠ **ALERT**

> Equine influenza is reported to affect donkeys severely. Consider antibiotic therapy early in the disease if there is any indication of secondary bronchopneumonia.

Testing for triglyceride levels will allow support of nutritional intake in order to avoid hyperlipaemia.

A vaccination programme should be considered to protect against current circulating strains.

Equine/Asinine Herpes virus (EHV) presents with similar clinical signs to those seen in horses and ponies. The donkey is susceptible to a similar range of herpes viruses and can develop respiratory, abortion and neurological signs in response to EHV 1 and 4, and coital exanthema following infection with EHV 3. The therapeutic and biosecurity measures for donkeys with EHV should be followed as per standard equine guidelines, but remember that severe respiratory infection may be complicated by hyperlipaemia.

⚠ **ALERT**

Stress and mixing with new donkeys may lead to recrudescence of clinical signs.

- Donkeys may also harbour host adapted asinine herpes virus which can cause a variety of syndromes including potentially contributing to fibrosing lung disease.

- Diagnosis of herpes virus infection can be by nasopharyngeal swab or by virus isolation from whole blood.

- Serological testing provides retrospective evidence of exposure, although high anti-complement levels in donkey serum may reduce the effectiveness of this test in some donkeys. A four-fold increase in titre between samples indicates evidence of infection.

Specific testing for asinine herpes virus is not readily available.

There is no data available on the effectiveness of herpes virus vaccination in donkeys.

Donkeys can be affected by both the commensal **Streptococcus equi subsp. zooepidemicus** and the pathogenic **Streptococcus equi subsp. equi.**

S. zooepidemicus is capable of causing severe empyema and chondroids in the guttural pouches.

As in horses and ponies, the carrier state involves harbouring the organism in the guttural pouches. Cases of nasal discharge should be investigated by culture and PCR using nasopharyngeal swabs/washes and endoscopy. Guttural pouch endoscopy in the donkey is not especially difficult or different to the horse and pony. It is advised to use the smallest nasopharyngeal swabs that your laboratory can supply and to carry out culture and PCR for S. equi.

The Animal Health Trust, Newmarket, UK can provide appropriately sized nasopharyngeal swabs for use in the donkey.

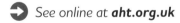 *See online at **aht.org.uk***

Commercially available serological tests for S. equi have not been validated in donkeys so should be interpreted with caution.

PARASITIC DISEASES

Dictyocaulus arnfieldii (lungworm). Donkeys do not often exhibit clinical signs of infection, yet may excrete large numbers of eggs in their faeces. Donkeys most at risk of developing disease related to high infection intensity are those that are geriatric and/or immunocompromised. The administration of corticosteroids or pituitary pars intermedia dysfunction appear to be correlated with higher lungworm burdens.

- Donkeys do not tend to cough when infected in the lower airways, unlike horses and ponies.

- Adult worms are found in the respiratory passages and eggs are coughed up and swallowed and passed out in the faeces. This is different to lungworms of other host species in which first stage larvae (L1) are usually detected in faecal samples.

- D. *arnfieldi* eggs hatch quickly, so diagnostic analysis should include the Baermann technique for L1 as well as examination for eggs by standard Faecal Egg Count (FEC) methods, particularly if samples are fresh and have been stored anaerobically.

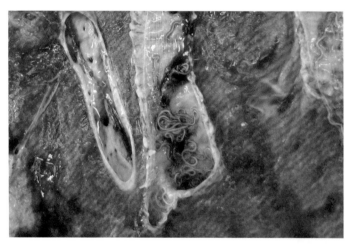

Adult lungworm in the respiratory passages.

➔ *See Chapter 11: Parasitology for more information.*

Parascaris equorum may cause lung damage and nasal discharge in younger donkeys as part of its migratory lifecycle.

Hydatidosis is seen in donkeys. It is diagnosed and treated as in horse and ponies.

OTHER CONDITIONS OF THE UPPER RESPIRATORY TRACT

Laryngeal paralysis in the donkey is more likely to be related to liver failure than to recurrent laryngeal neuropathy.

Soft palate displacements may be detected at endoscopy. They will not be detected by identification of abnormal noises when ridden at speed as in horses and ponies.

Dental disease may be associated with, or lead to, **Sinus disease**, especially in geriatric donkeys.

Empyema of the guttural pouch may follow infection with *S. equi* and *S. zooepidemicus*. It is diagnosed and treated as in horses and ponies.

Guttural pouch mycosis (GPM) can occur in the donkey, but is very infrequent, possibly due to the variation in the carotid arterial tree anatomy. However, where it has been reported in the donkey, epistaxis together with acute dyspnoea was noted, the dyspnoea relating to the narrow donkey nasopharynx and other subtle anatomical variations.

Tracheal collapse is usually seen in older donkeys due to age-related degeneration of the tracheal rings or cartilage, or secondary to a condition that causes increased inspiratory effort such as pulmonary fibrosis.

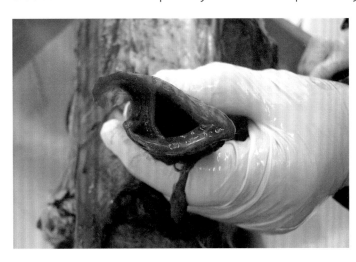

Tracheal collapse – note marked narrowing of airway.

Note that:

- Clinical signs include harsh stertorous or honking sounds, dyspnoea and a chronic cough.

- Vibrations may be felt on palpation of the trachea over the collapsed area.

- The distal cervical and rostral thoracic regions of the trachea contain the most dorso-ventrally flattened rings where there is the highest incidence of collapse.

- Radiography or endoscopy can confirm the diagnosis. Endoscopy is poorly tolerated in the severely affected or acute cases.

Treatment of any underlying lung disease, maintenance of a dust-free environment, and management of an acute crisis with steroids (inhaled or systemic) atropine and diuretics can be attempted, but in severe cases euthanasia is usually the only option.

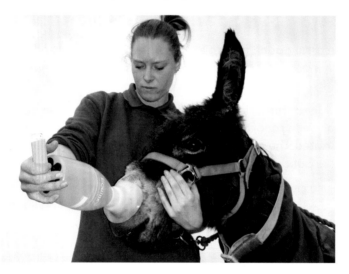

Use of inhaled medication in a donkey.

OTHER CONDITIONS OF THE LOWER RESPIRATORY TRACT

⚠ **ALERT**

The donkey may have severe disease before diagnosis due to the lack of ridden work and an insensitive cough reflex.

Recurrent airway obstruction is diagnosed and treated as in horses and ponies, but note:

- Most donkeys tolerate inhalation therapy well.

- Check the medical history for laminitis and Equine Metabolic Syndrome (EMS) and be aware of the potential risks of using long-term steroid therapy in any high-risk or obese donkey.

- Try to use a low calorie, donkey short chopped forage product to avoid dusty straw.

➜ *See online at **thedonkeysanctuary.org.uk/for-professionals** for more information on feeding the donkey with respiratory conditions.*

Pulmonary fibrosis is a chronic interstitial fibrosing lung disease which has been described in donkeys in the UK and USA. The aetiology is unknown, but equine/asinine herpes viruses have been isolated from some cases in both donkeys and horses. Late presentation of a donkey showing an advanced stage of the disease is typical. Note that:

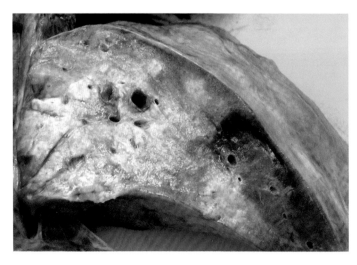

Typical peribronchial fibrosis.

- Lesions can be sub-pleural or fibrosis can extend through the interstitial lung tissue.

- Clinical signs include increased respiratory effort (dyspnoea) on both inspiration and expiration.

- Auscultation of the lung field may reveal areas where there is complete absence of sounds as the lung is now fibrotic, and areas where adventitious wheezes and crackles are present in hyper-inflated or constricted small airways.

- Radiography could aid diagnosis.

- There may be episodes of pyrexia and nasal discharge if secondary infections occur.

Treatment is palliative, with good management and judicious use of bronchodilators, steroids, anti-inflammatories and antibiotics. Some reports suggest that anti-viral medications may be of use in cases that are caught at the early stages and with a known viral aetiology.

Pulmonary neoplasia has a low incidence, reported as 0.4% in one study (Thiemann 2012). However, the donkey is often kept until an advanced age and thoracic neoplasia should be considered as a differential diagnosis for chronic cases of respiratory disease. Clinical signs may include dullness, pyrexia, weight loss and ventral oedema in addition to tachypnoea and dyspnoea. In most cases diagnosis is likely to be made at post-mortem examination.

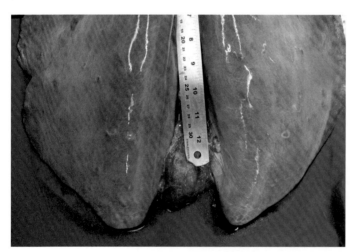

Right and left lung; multifocal, up to 0.5cm in diameter, round, white, firm masses within the lung parenchyma (metastatic neoplasia).

PREVENTION

The experience of The Donkey Sanctuary is that a high proportion of donkeys receive inadequate preventative healthcare. This is likely to increase the incidence of diseases of the respiratory system and this is a significant cause of morbidity and mortality and can have implications for the welfare of the donkey.

Prevention is important and a good programme of vaccination and surveillance, along with biosecurity measures, should be in place. Note that:

- Donkeys should be vaccinated against equine respiratory diseases using standard equine protocols. In most cases there will not be vaccines licensed for donkeys, or data as to their efficacy.

- Surveillance, especially the screening of new donkeys, can reduce the risk of infection.

⚠ **ALERT**

Donkeys can be subclinical carriers of equine and asinine herpes virus, which can recrudesce in response to stress.

- Due to the existence of the carrier state with both herpes viruses and *S. equi*, new donkeys introduced to a group or premises with other equines should undergo standard isolation procedures.

- Guttural pouch washes/nasopharyngeal swabs should be taken to check for *S. equi*, It is advised to use the smallest nasopharyngeal swabs that your laboratory can supply and to carry out culture and PCR for *S. equi*.

- Commercially available serological tests for *S. equi* have not been validated in donkeys so should be interpreted with caution.

Remember that donkeys have a relatively insensitive cough reflex so it is important not to rely on clinical signs alone when screening new arrivals for respiratory disease. Check the temperature and inflammatory markers, including white cell counts and ratios and acute phase proteins. Use nasopharyngeal swabs and guttural pouch washes.

Lungworm is hard to eradicate from paddocks. Isolate, test and treat new arrivals before they share pasture with horses and ponies.

🐴 MULES AND HINNIES

There is limited information or evidence available for respiratory conditions in mules and therefore nothing to add that is specific to the mule.

ℹ️ FURTHER INFORMATION

Factsheets, research and detailed information can be found online at:
thedonkeysanctuary.org.uk/for-professionals

Kleiboeker, S.B., Schommer, S.K., Johnson, P.J., Ehlers, B., Turnquist, S.E., Boucher, M. and Kreeger, J.M. (2002) Association of two newly recognized herpes viruses with interstitial pneumonia in donkeys *(Equus asinus). J. Vet. Diag. Invest.* 14, 273—280.

Powell, R.J., du Toit, N., Burden, F.A. and Dixon, P.M. (2009) Morphological study of tracheal shape in donkeys with and without tracheal obstruction. *Equine Vet. J.* 42, 136—141.

Thiemann, A.K. (2012) Respiratory disease in the donkey. *Equine Vet Education.* 2012; 9: 469—478.

5. THE NERVOUS SYSTEM

Although many of the conditions of the nervous system in donkeys are very similar to those in horses and ponies, there are some subtle differences in presenting signs and requirements for examination. As with other conditions in donkeys, it is very important to monitor the animal regularly for hyperlipaemia, which may be secondary to a neurological condition.

CLINICAL EXAMINATION

DIAGNOSTIC PROCEDURES

CONDITIONS

TREATMENT

- Differentiating between the ataxic donkey and one that is lame can be challenging.

- The stoic donkey may show a greater tolerance to menace testing and any lack of reaction should be interpreted with caution.

CLINICAL EXAMINATION

Following a full clinical examination, the neurological examination of the donkey should be performed systematically in the same way as in horses and ponies, assessing mentation, posture, cranial nerve activity, gait, strength and reflexes.

Mentation

Given that donkeys are frequently unaccustomed to veterinary examination, the owner's observations about any changes in behaviour can be very valuable. The donkey is best observed undisturbed in a relaxed, preferably normal environment, in order to identify subtle abnormalities while at rest.

Posture

Neurological abnormalities may lead to a lower head position in the donkey. However, care should be taken because systemic disease leading to pyrexia, dullness or pain may also cause a similar postural change.

Cranial nerve activity

A methodical cranial nerve examination should show the same responses as in the horse and pony.

Note that:

- The stoic donkey may show a greater tolerance to menace testing and this test should be repeated before the donkey is diagnosed with a lack of menace response.

- A true lack of menace response should lead the clinician to perform an ophthalmic examination and a sight test to distinguish blindness from facial nerve dysfunction.

- Blindfolding will enable identification of vestibular disease that has been compensated for by visual orientation, because the donkey will develop a head tilt or ataxia once vision is obscured.

Gait

Differentiating between the ataxic donkey and one with orthopaedic gait abnormalities can be challenging.

Dynamic assessment is complicated due to the donkey's 'freeze' response to fearful situations, the wide range of conformational and gait abnormalities observed in this species, and lack of training to walk and trot on a loose rein.

Note that:

- The ataxic donkey may show an irregularly-irregular gait pattern, whereas a lameness or conformational gait abnormality will generally exhibit a consistent abnormal limb placement.

- A 'pacing' gait (two-beat, lateral movement at the same speed as a walk) may indicate spinal cord disease.

> ⚠ **ALERT**
>
> The risk of secondary hyperlipaemia should always be considered during treatment of a primary neurological condition.

Strength

The donkey's age and workload should be taken into account when assessing strength. This can vary significantly between young working animals and elderly companion donkeys.

Reflexes

Reflexes are examined and interpreted in the same way as in horses and ponies. However, the response, or lack of response, to the menace test must be interpreted with caution.

DIAGNOSTIC PROCEDURES

Laboratory diagnosis

Full haematology and biochemistry is indicated in the neurological work up, including triglycerides and inflammatory markers.

Serum amyloid A is a more sensitive marker of inflammation than fibrinogen. It responds within 24 hours of acute inflammation and is a useful tool to grade the level of inflammation and to monitor progress of an inflammatory response.

When assessing vitamin E levels remember that they may vary during the day. A more accurate representation of vitamin E status may be gained by taking 3 samples over a 24 hour period rather than a single sample.

The painful, inappetent or dysphagic donkey is at high risk of developing hyperlipaemia. Blood samples should be monitored regularly throughout the course of treatment of the neurological condition, to prevent or diagnose secondary hyperlipaemia.

Rectal examination

Palpation of internal structures can be performed in most donkeys despite their smaller size in relation to horses and ponies. Most donkeys tolerate the procedure well but some may require sedation. Good lubrication will aid the procedure and spasmolytic medication can be used where appropriate to facilitate the examination – for example, hyoscine butylbromide at 0.3mg/kg IV (Buscopan 20mg/ml).

Rectal examination will be most valuable in those animals presenting with hindlimb ataxia or cauda equina syndrome, with specific attention paid to the size of the bladder, vertebral palpation and iliac artery pulsation.

Radiography

Spinal radiographs may be more useful than in the horse, pony or mule due to the smaller size of most donkeys. The techniques are the same as in horses and ponies.

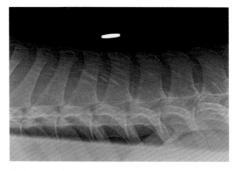

Cerebrospinal fluid (CSF) collection

CSF can be collected using the same landmarks as in the horse and pony – via the lumbosacral space in the conscious donkey or the atlanto-occipital space in the anaesthetised animal or cadaver.

Spinal radiograph of the donkey.

CONDITIONS

The differential diagnoses for neurological symptoms in the donkey are generally the same as in the horse and pony.

Notable differences are seen:

- where vaccination or prophylaxis is rarely used in the donkey. This is particularly relevant to infections such as tetanus, or

- where the weight of the donkey is estimated incorrectly and a drug overdose is given.

Infectious diseases

Many diseases in donkeys show similar signs and require similar treatment to those in horses and ponies.

 See Chapter 10: Infectious Diseases for more information.

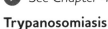

Be aware of zoonotic implications, where relevant, and take precautions.

Herpes virus infection

Until recently equine herpes virus 1 (EHV 1) was not thought to cause a neurological syndrome in the donkey and donkeys were thought to be silent reservoirs of the virus. Cases of equine herpes virus 1 myeloencephalopathy in the donkey have been reported as showing similar clinical signs to horses and ponies with EHV 1 infection. The disease showed a rapid progression with high mortality.

An additional case report identified a donkey with transient neurological symptoms associated with a gamma herpesvirus similar to Asinine herpes virus 5, normally implicated in interstitial pneumonia.

 See Chapter 4: The Respiratory System for more information.

Trypanosomiasis

Neurological symptoms are seen in the donkey and recent studies in Gambia show an increasing incidence of the neurological form. The disease is often fatal, and, in donkeys, clinical signs are associated with deteriorating cerebral function and cranial nerve abnormalities with diffuse lymphocytic-plasmacytic meningo–encephalomyelitis.

Rabies

Working donkeys become infected by rabies from the bites of infected carnivores, usually dogs, jackals, hyenas or foxes. They are at risk because they are often kept outside at night or allowed to wander freely.

Note that:

- Reports from Latin America show that donkeys are more likely to be attacked by vampire bats than horses and ponies and vampire bat-transmitted rabies in donkeys has been reported in Mexico.

- Donkeys may show vague, non-specific signs, such as depression, anorexia and colic, at an early stage of the disease.

- Apparent oesophageal obstruction ('choke') is reported as a common initial presenting sign.

- 'Furious' (neurological) signs are common in the advanced stage of the disease, and are characterised by aggressive behaviours such as trying to bite other animals or handlers, baring teeth, teeth grinding, self-mutilation, and eating foreign bodies.

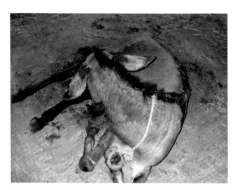 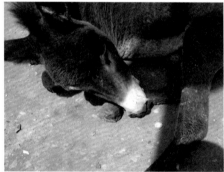

Rabid donkeys mutilating themselves.

- Donkeys may die within a few days of the onset of clinical signs. However, progression can be slower (up to two weeks) in some cases.

Tetanus

Tetanus is reported to be a significant cause of death among working donkeys, mules, horses and ponies. There is an increased risk of disease in the donkey as many animals do not have an effective vaccination programme.

⚠ **ALERT**

Tetanus prophylaxis is an important consideration when treating any wound because few donkeys are vaccinated.

Clinical signs result from hypertonicity and cranial nerve defects, and are similar to those seen in horses and ponies.

Causes and increased risk of infection commonly arise from:

- penetrating foot injuries

- wounds from poor fitting harnesses and tack

- wounds that are not identified at an early stage due to the thick coat of the donkey and the lack of regular grooming and management practices that would aid detection.

Diagnosis and treatment is as in horses and ponies.

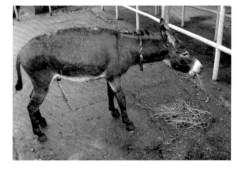

Donkey with typical generalised tetany and lock jaw.

Drug toxicity

Accurate weight estimation is essential for calculating drug dosages. Difficulties in accurately estimating the weight of a donkey can lead to overdosing and toxicity.

⚠ **ALERT**

Accurate weight estimation is essential. Horse and pony weigh tapes are not suitable for the donkey.

The donkey specific nomogram may be used to estimate the weight of an animal.

➜ *See Appendix 2 for The Donkey Sanctuary Weight Estimator.*

A weigh tape has been developed specifically for the donkey. This is suitable for estimating the weight of a donkey whilst horse and pony weigh tapes are not.

➜ *See online at* **www.donkeyweightape.com** *for a donkey specific weigh tape.*

Examples of drug toxicity presenting with neurological signs are:

- Aminoglycoside - vestibulocochlear nerve defects

- Ivermectin - blindness.

- Moxidectin- seizures

- Enrofloxacin- seizures

TREATMENT

Treatment and management of neurological conditions in the donkey follow the same principles as in the horse and pony.

Donkeys may tolerate periods of recumbency better than horses and ponies due to their smaller size and weight. As with other species, recumbent donkeys should be placed on soft bedding (a mattress or the padded floor of an induction box with thick bedding are most appropriate) and they should be turned every 2—6 hours even if able to maintain sternal recumbency. Legs can be wrapped with soft bandages, and head bumpers can be fitted to prevent further head trauma in the ataxic or recumbent patient.

🐎 MULES AND HINNIES

There is limited information or evidence available for neurological conditions in mules and therefore nothing to add that is specific to the mule.

ⓘ FURTHER INFORMATION

Factsheets, research and detailed information can be found online at: **thedonkeysanctuary.org.uk/for-professionals**

The Working Equid Veterinary Manual: **thebrooke.org/for-professionals/ working-equid-veterinary-manual**

Furr, M. and Reed, S. (2008) Equine Neurology. 1st Edition. Blackwell Publishing Ltd.

Mayhew, I.G., Brewer B.D., Reinhard, M.K. et al (1984). Verminous (Strongylus vulgaris) myelitis in a donkey. *Cornell Vet* 74: 30—7.

Reed, S.M., Bayly, W.M. and Sellon, D.C. (2003) Equine Internal Medicine. 2nd Edition. Saunders.

Vengust, M., Wen, X. and Bienzle, D. (2008) Herpesvirus associated neurological disease in a donkey. *J Vet Diagn Invest* 20: 820—823.

Negussie, H., Gizaw, D., Tessema, T.S. and Nauwynck, H.J. (2017) Equine Herpesvirus-1 Myeloencephalopathy, an emerging threat of working equids in Ethiopia. *Transboundary and Emerging Diseases*. 64: 389—397.

6. THE REPRODUCTIVE SYSTEM

While donkey reproduction and castration can be approached in a similar way to horses and ponies there are important differences to note.

Sexual behaviour is often more exaggerated in the donkey and stallion like behaviour may persist in the male donkey after castration. It is recommended that all male donkeys are castrated unless they are intended for breeding, and that this is carried out between 6 and 18 months.

MANAGEMENT OF REPRODUCTION

PREGNANCY

PARTURITION

COMMON CONDITIONS

CASTRATION

KEY POINTS

- Castration will avoid unwanted pregnancies and reduce aggressive behaviour. It is therefore recommended that all male donkeys are castrated if they have no breeding use.

- The optimum age for castration is 6—18 months.

- It is strongly recommended that all donkeys over four years old or with large and well-developed testicles are castrated using the inguinal approach.

- Ligation of the testicular artery is mandatory when castrating donkeys.

- Length of gestation is variable in the donkey, with a range of 11—14.5 months.

The donkey has several anatomical differences to the horse and pony:

- The ligament of the salpinx is wider than in mares, covering the lateral aspect of the ovary.

- The position of the ovaries is slightly further cranial than in mares.

- The tips of the uterine horns are situated on a level with the fifth lumbar vertebra and the ovaries lie ventral to the fourth and fifth lumbar vertebra.

- Tortuous longitudinal folds are found within the cervical channel. The asinine cervix is rather long, small and tight.

- The male donkey has proportionally larger reproductive organs and associated vasculature.

Specific characteristics of the female reproductive cycle include:

- Females start cycling regularly between 10 and 22 months old.

- The duration of dioestrus is approximately 18 days (16—20 days).

- Interoestrus intervals are approximately 24 days (20—26 days).

- Oestrus duration is variable, around six days (2—10 days).

- Older females tend to show longer interovulatory intervals.

During oestrus female donkeys display a variety of behaviours that include mounting, herding, chasing other females, mouth clapping, winking (repeated exposure of the clitoris), raising the tail, urination, posturing (ie abducted rear legs, arched tail, tipped pelvis, and lowered perineal area), and standing to be mounted.

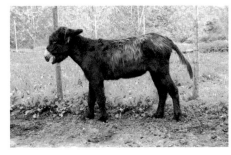

A female donkey in oestrus.

During dioestrus females will show a lack of interest in the male. They typically hold their tail down between the hind legs and refuse the male by moving away or kicking.

The average size of the dominant follicle at the onset of oestrus is 25mm. The maximum follicular diameter in single ovulations prior to ovulation is 41mm. Ovulation generally occurs less than 15 hours before the end of oestrus. Oestrus behaviour continues for a variable period after ovulation.

Double ovulations may occur more frequently than in horses and ponies, ranging from 5—70%, with a high individual repeatability. Prevalence of multiple ovulations seems to be positively affected by body condition.

Reproductive function appears less affected by season in donkeys. A relatively high number of donkeys have regular oestrous cycles throughout the year, although seasonal anoestrus may occur. Females with a lower body score condition may enter anoestrus.

Foaling before four years old may be associated with a higher mortality of the foal and/or dam.

Specific characteristics of the male donkey sexual behaviour include:

• Puberty in the male donkey occurs between 16 and 20 months old.

• Sexual maturity is attained at around three years old.

• Mating will normally take longer in the donkey than in the horse and pony.

It is usual for several periods of sexual interaction, separated by periods of male withdrawal from the female. It is normal for the male donkey to mount several times without erection and this behaviour should not be discouraged because it will allow the male to become fully aroused.

There may be a point during the courtship when the male appears to lose interest in the female and backs off a few metres prior to full erection and mating.

Mount, coitus and ejaculation is usually attained after 15 to 30 minutes, and this process should not be hurried.

> ⚠ **ALERT**
>
> Males can be very aggressive. This is exacerbated by the presence of competing males and females in season. Muzzling may be necessary.

> ℹ **INFORMATION**
>
> **Semen constitution**
> * Volume: 30—150ml
> * Concentration: 100×10^6—400×10^6/ml

MANAGEMENT OF REPRODUCTION

The oestrous cycle of the female donkey can be manipulated in the same way as in horses and ponies.

Semen from the male donkey can be collected using the same artificial vaginas as those used for stallions. The presence of a female in heat is generally necessary to attain erection and ejaculation, even when using a dummy.

Male donkeys may require some time to achieve full erection, with repeated mounting prior to successful ejaculation.

Low sperm survival, low conception rate with frozen semen, and the low survival of embryos after transfer to recipients have been noted when using artificial insemination and embryo transfer.

Contraception may be appropriate in some feral populations. Control methods such as the use of porcine zona pellucida immunocontraception, gonadotropin-releasing hormone, oocyte-specific growth factors, bone morphogenetic protein 15 (BMP15), or an intrauterine device may be considered. Information or evidence for their use in donkeys is limited.

PREGNANCY

Gestation is longer and with greater variability than in horses and ponies. The average length is usually between 365 and 376 days but it can range between 11 and 14.5 months.

The incidence of twin foaling at full gestation is reportedly higher than in horses and ponies.

Diagnosis of pregnancy

Transrectal ultrasound can be carried out as early as 10 days after ovulation when embryonic vesicles (EV) may be detected. The optimal time for early pregnancy diagnosis is 14 days after ovulation.

Transrectal palpation can be performed from day 40.

Oestrone sulphate plasma concentrations can also be used. Concentrations are reported to increase from week 15, remain greater than 500ng/mL between weeks 18 and 33, and then decrease thereafter, reaching mean values of less than 100ng/mL from week 42.

The Cuboni reaction, a urine test based on the reaction of oestrogens.

Stages of foetal development detectable by ultrasound:

Characteristic	Days of gestation Mean / Range	Diameter (mm)
EV detection	11.5 (10—14)	6.5
EV fixation	18 (16—20)	
EV loss of spherical shape	19 (18—20)	
Embryo detection	22 (20—24	
Heart beat detection	25 (24—26)	
Allantoic sac detection	27 (26—28)	
Umbilical cord detection	46 (45—47)	
Sex determination TAU (start)	22 weeks	
Sex determination TAU (best)	35—38 weeks	
Sex determination TAU (end)	42 weeks	
Transrectal ultrasound (TRU)	56 - 64	
Chest / thorax detection	60 (54—64)	17.2
Stomach detection	66.5 (60—71)	
Eye orbit detection	81 (71—96)	6.7
Aorta detection	94.5 (79—109)	3.5

Pregnancy termination

Twin pregnancies may be more common in donkeys than in horses and ponies. Twin pregnancies may be higher in certain breeds, certain familial lines and certain individuals. Manual reduction of one of the EV's is preferably done on days 14—15 and successful termination confirmed before day 35.

Care in pregnancy

Pregnant females should be vaccinated following recommended equine guidelines.

Prior to foaling, preventive measures for the control of parasites should be undertaken, including a plan for appropriate pasture management during and after pregnancy.

Female body condition should be regularly assessed and feed adjusted appropriately.

 See chapter 18: Nutrition for more information about nutrition in pregnancy.

PARTURITION

Due to variability in the length of gestation, all preparation and planning for regular observation and potential assistance must be in place before 11 months gestation.

Typically, the udder starts developing four to six weeks prior to foaling, often with oedema developing that may only be obvious in the last days of pregnancy. A ventral oedema can develop cranial to the udder. Softening of the pelvic ligaments begins in the last three to four weeks, and terminally the belly looks more pendulous and the teats finally develop.

When secretion is present, the visual examination of a few drops stripped from the teats can be used to estimate when foaling will occur. The secretion starts as clear and watery, progresses to cloudy, then becomes yellow-tinged and sticky, finally looking like opaque white milk in the last 24 to 48 hours.

Hygiene precautions should be taken to prevent mastitis.

Electrolyte levels in the mammary secretions can be used to predict foaling:

- A sodium: potassium ratio of less than 1 is indicative of foaling occurring in the next 24 to 48 hours.

- Calcium levels can also be used but are less reliable.

In the last days to hours before foaling, the cervical seal liquefies with a mucoid discharge. In the last 24 hours females become more isolated. The vulva becomes longer, flatter and increasingly flaccid. In the majority of cases parturition occurs at night.

First, second and third stage labour generally progress as in horses and ponies and should be managed accordingly.

Post-partum

Female donkeys may have a higher tendency to exhibit foal heat than horses and ponies, with higher pregnancy rates. Breeding at the foal heat or first oestrous cycles post-partum is a viable possibility.

A clear and odourless vaginal discharge is normal up to one week post-partum, and some intrauterine fluid may still be present after two weeks.

COMMON CONDITIONS

> ⚠ **ALERT**
>
> Overweight female donkeys are at particular risk of hyperlipaemia during pregnancy and lactation.

Infectious conditions

All equine infectious reproductive diseases may affect donkeys.

The South African strain of Equine Viral Arteritis (EVA) is common among South African donkeys. It was shown to have low pathogenicity in both species, including pregnant mares, and to be poorly transmissible to horses. This EVA variant seems to be very distinct from that found in equids in Europe and North America.

➡ *See Chapter 10: Infectious Diseases for more information.*

Donkeys may be infected with *Taylorella asinigenitalis* (currently considered not pathogenic). This may complicate diagnosis when screening for *T. equigenitalis*.

Congenital disorders have been reported – for example, cervical hypoplasia and persistent hymen in the Burro de Miranda breed of donkey.

Mastitis and metritis may be more frequently seen in working donkeys kept in unsanitary environments. Both conditions are treated and managed as in horses and ponies.

Ovulation fossa inclusion cysts are reported in female donkeys. A genetic predisposition is suspected in the Burro de Miranda breed. Ovaries up to 25cm in diameter have been found due to the presence of these cysts. Generally, cysts are multiple, ranging from 2—110mm in diameter, and may affect both ovaries. Most cases are benign incidental findings. Abdominal pain is sometimes identified, in which case drainage or excision is required.

CASTRATION

Castration is recommended to prevent aggression and unwanted pregnancies.

The optimum age for castration is 6–18 months.

> ⚠ **ALERT**
>
> **There is an increased risk of haemorrhage from all tissues in the donkey. The testicular arteries within the spermatic cord must be ligated.**

There are important specific considerations to take into account when planning to castrate a donkey:

- There are two different techniques for castration: closed castration (using a scrotal approach) and an inguinal approach. Choice will depend on the age and size of the stallion:

  - If the donkey is less than two years old and both testicles have descended, closed castration using the scrotal approach should be used.

  - If the donkey is over four years old or over 150kg and the testicles large and well developed, the inguinal approach is strongly recommended in order to reduce post-operative complications. Inguinal castration is best performed in a dedicated equine operating environment.

  - If the donkey is between two and four years old and under 150kg, a decision should be made based on the size of the testicles. In most cases the scrotal approach will be appropriate.

- There is an increased risk of haemorrhage in the donkey due to well developed blood vessels. A ligature around the vaginal tunic, including the testicular artery, is therefore essential.

- There may be a significant amount of scrotal and inguinal fat even in slim donkeys. The fat may need to be trimmed to avoid prolapsing from the open scrotal incision.

- The aforementioned points and the diminutive size of the donkey make castration a procedure best done under general anaesthesia.

- Peri-operative and post-operative analgesia is mandatory.

- The stoic nature of the donkey can result in post-operative problems being overlooked.

➡ *See Chapter 16: Sedation, Anaesthesia and Analgesia for more information.*

> ⚠ **ALERT**
>
> Keep stress and pain to a minimum to reduce the risk of hyperlipaemia.

Pre-anaesthetic preparation and anaesthesia

It is essential to plan appropriately, ensuring that all drugs and equipment, including those for emergency use, are available and in good order.

➡ See Chapter 16: Sedation, Anaesthesia and Analgesia for more information.

> ⚠ **ALERT**
>
> Consider the technique to be used – closed scrotal approach or inguinal approach – according to the age and size of the donkey.

Some important points to remember when anaesthetising the donkey are:

- Preparation and planning are important and consideration of the companion donkey is essential.

- Be aware of the risks of peri-operative hyperlipaemia, especially as a result of stress, pain, disease or pre-anaesthetic starvation.

- Be aware of the risk of underlying disease that may be missed due to the stoic nature of the donkey. Pre-operative examination is essential and blood tests may be considered advisable.

- Remember that weight estimation is different for donkeys than for horses and ponies and is important for calculating drug dosages.

- Check the vaccination status of the donkey for tetanus; it may be necessary to administer prophylaxis.

- Give peri-operative non-steroidal analgesia, either phenylbutazone or flunixin meglumine, twice daily.

Closed scrotal approach

This is recommended for colts and less mature stallions. It is not recommended for stallions over four years old or with well-developed testicles because of the greater risk of post-operative complications.

When using the closed scrotal approach:

- Operate under general anaesthesia, with the donkey in lateral recumbency.

- Have the upper hind leg tied or held up by an assistant standing spine-side if in the field.

- It is vital to close clip and use thorough surgical disinfection due to the ligature placement.

- Intra-testicular local anaesthetic can be used for pain relief and to facilitate anaesthesia. Inject after the initial skin preparation using 10—15mls of lignocaine at the junction between each cord and testicle, avoiding blood vessels.

- Make two parallel sharp incisions through the skin of the scrotum down to the *tunica vaginalis communis*. Ensure they are positioned at the most dependant point when the donkey stands, and are sufficiently long to get the testicle out without excessive force.

- Start with the lower testicle.

> ⚠ **ALERT**
>
> **Even a slim donkey can have a considerable amount of scrotal fat. Care must be taken to ensure the fat does not prolapse from the wound.**

- Remove fat using a dry gauze swab or clamp and cut, being aware of rupturing any blood vessels but removing anything that might prolapse from the wound.

- The cremaster muscle can be left in place because the ligature will usually cut through when tightened and the muscle may haemorrhage if transected sharply.

- Good clean exposure of the spermatic cord enables the optimal ligation site to be identified. A second pair of hands scrubbed in can assist with gentle retraction of the testicle as the ligature is placed.

- Crushing the cord prior to laying the ligature allows better security and haemostasis.

- Ligate using five metric braided absorbable suture material.

- Experience suggests that a constrictor ligature with an additional four single throws is effective, staying tight and avoiding the need to transfix the ligature.

The constrictor ligature:

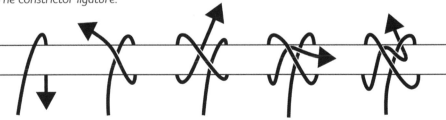

1. Place working end over cord,
2. cross over the static end,
3. go round the back and through again,
4. take the working end and go over the first loop,
5. then under towards the middle and pull up tight.

- The spermatic cord should be transected by crush and cut or emasculators 1cm below the ligature.

- Leave tissue forceps attached to the stump to check for bleeding before releasing.

- Once both testicles have been resected, carefully excise tissue which may prolapse from the wound.

Inguinal approach

The inguinal approach is recommended for mature or large male donkeys, generally over four years of age. The procedure is carried out in the same way as for horses and ponies. It should only be performed in a dedicated equine operating environment.

Post-operative care

This should include:

- Hose with cold water for 5—10 minutes once or twice daily (directing water to the top of the scrotum, not directly into the open incisions where the scrotal approach has been used).

- Carry out in hand walking exercise.

- Allow access to a clean exercise yard or paddock rather than limiting to stable rest.

- Monitor appetite and demeanour closely for signs of discomfort or stress. Urgent veterinary attention is required if the donkey is inappetent, due to the risk of hyperlipaemia.

Post-operative complications are treated and managed as in horses and ponies. Prolapse of fat from the wound is commonly seen when this has not been adequately removed during surgery.

Some stallion like behaviour may persist for extended periods post castration, notably in more mature and sexually active animals.

🐴 MULES AND HINNIES

Even though they are sterile, it is advisable to castrate stallion mules to minimise aggressive behaviour.

ℹ️ FURTHER INFORMATION

Factsheets, research and detailed information can be found online at: **thedonkeysanctuary.org.uk/for-professionals**

The Working Equid Veterinary Manual: **thebrooke.org/for-professionals/ working-equid-veterinary-manual**

Bonelli, F., Rota, A., Corazza, M., Serio, D., & Sgorbini, M. (2016). Hematological and biochemical findings in pregnant, postfoaling, and lactating jennies. *Theriogenology*, 85(7), 1233–1238.

Carluccio, A., De Amicis, I., Panzani, S., Tosi, U., Faustini, M., & Veronesi, M. (2008). Electrolytes Changes in Mammary Secretions Before Foaling in Jennies. Reproduction in Domestic Animals, 43(2), 162–165.

Conceição JC, Freitas Neto LM, Aguiar Filho CR, Araújo GHM, Oliveira JV, Bartolomeu CC, Oba E, Meira C (2009) Ultrasound evaluation of ovarian follicular dynamics in Jennies (Equus asinus) during the estrous cycle. *Medicina Veterinária* 3, 7-14.

Crisci, A., Rota, A., Panzani, D., Sgorbini, M., Ousey, J. C., & Camillo, F. (2014). Clinical, ultrasonographic, and endocrinological studies on donkey pregnancy. *Theriogenology*, 81(2), 275–283.

Kalender H, Aslan S, Schwarzenberger F, Maral NE, Izgur H, Handler J, Findik M (2012) Uterine involution, follicle development and concentrations of plasma progesterone, 20α-OH-progesterone and total estrogen levels during the postpartum period in Anatolian donkeys. KAFKAS UNIVERSITESI *Veteriner Fakultesi Dergisi* 18, 929-933.

Quaresma, M., & Payan-Carreira, R. (2015). Characterization of the estrous cycle of Asinina de Miranda jennies (Equus asinus). *Theriogenology*, 83(4), 616–624.

Quaresma, M., Payan-Carreira, R., Pires, M. dos A., & Edwards, J. F. (2011). Bilateral Ovulation Fossa Inclusion Cysts in Miranda Jennets. *Journal of Comparative Pathology*, 145(4), 367–372.

Quaresma, M., Payan-Carreira, R., & Silva, S. R. (2013). Relationship between ultrasound measurements of body fat reserves and body condition score in female donkeys. *The Veterinary Journal*, 197(2), 329–334.

Sprayson, T., & Thiemann, A. (2007). Clinical approach to castration in the donkey. *In Practice*, 29(9), 526–531.

Vincenzetti, S., Polidori, P., Mariani, P., Cammertoni, N., Fantuz, F., & Vita, A. (2008). Donkey's milk protein fractions characterization. *Food Chemistry*, 106(2), 640–649.

7. HYPERLIPAEMIA AND THE ENDOCRINE SYSTEM

Donkeys are particularly susceptible to hyperlipaemia. It can progress rapidly and is often life threatening. Prompt diagnosis and treatment is required to improve the outcome. If the donkey is managed correctly, with an appropriate diet and regular routine preventative healthcare, this risk can be minimised.

It is important to recognise circumstances that increase the risk of hyperlipaemia, such as pregnancy and lactation, and ensure that dietary requirements are met during these periods. Likewise, when treating a donkey for any condition that is likely to be painful or affect appetite, secondary hyperlipaemia needs to be considered. When stressful circumstances can't be avoided extra attention needs to be paid to appetite, and any reduction should warrant early intervention.

Pituitary pars intermedia dysfunction (PPID, also known as Cushing's disease) and Equine Metabolic Syndrome (EMS) are both recognised in donkeys. There are some donkey specifics that are of note in both conditions.

Laminitis may be the only clinical indicator of either PPID or EMS.

HYPERLIPAEMIA

PITUITARY PARS INTERMEDIA DYSFUNCTION (PPID)

EQUINE METABOLIC SYNDROME (EMS)

PREVENTION

KEY POINTS

- Early intervention to restore a positive energy balance even before triglyceride values are known greatly increases the chance of survival.

- Hyperlipaemia is often secondary to concurrent disease, so triglycerides should be checked as part of the diagnostic work up.

- Triglyceride levels should be checked in all inappetent donkeys.

- Survival is more likely if triglycerides are less than 10 mmol/l.

- Aggressive therapy is required if triglycerides exceed 10 mmol/l.

Donkey specific reference ranges for ACTH and insulin have been developed by The Donkey Sanctuary. These are for donkeys aged 3-20 years of age and the ACTH ranges are seasonally adjusted.

ⓘ INFORMATION

ACTH and insulin reference ranges for the adult donkey		
Insulin (uIU/ml)	0 - 15.1	
ACTH (pg/ml)	2.7 - 30.4	in November – June
	9.0 - 49.1	in July – October
Range was set up using the **TOSOH AIA-360 analyser.**		

HYPERLIPAEMIA

The pathophysiological process is triggered in response to a negative energy balance resulting in mobilisation of fats from adipose tissue. Although this is a normal response to a fasting state, in hyperlipaemia the rate of lipolysis exceeds the rate of uptake of triglycerides into peripheral tissue for use as an energy substrate. The accumulation of plasma triglycerides results in fatty infiltration of organs such as the liver, pancreas and kidneys, which can in turn, lead to multiple organ failure.

Pathophysiology

The mobilisation of fats from adipose tissue is under hormonal control but can also be influenced by cytokines such as granulocyte macrophage colony stimulating factor (GM-CSF) and tumour necrosis factor α (TNF-α), which are produced in inflammatory diseases. Stimulation of β-receptors by catecholamines and release of cortisol also promote lipolysis.

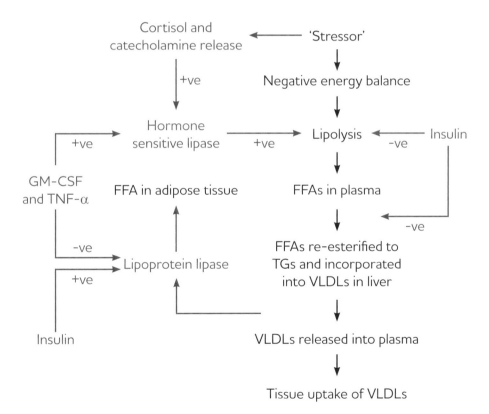

Pathway for mobilisation of fats stored in adipose tissue for use as an energy source in peripheral tissues. (FFA = free fatty acids, VLDL = very low density lipoprotein, TG = triglyceride).

Note that:

- Any condition or circumstance that reduces appetite will stimulate lipolysis.

- Donkeys are inherently insulin resistant and obesity predisposes to insulin resistance. Insulin resistance facilitates lipolysis.

- Stress results in the release of cortisol and catecholamines, which promote lipolysis.

- Cytokines promote lipolysis and inhibit very low density lipoprotein (VLDL) clearance by inhibiting lipoprotein lipase-induced uptake into adipose tissue. The resultant imbalance between release of fatty acids and uptake into peripheral tissue causes hyperlipaemia.

Epidemiology

Hyperlipaemia is unlikely to occur in the absence of a predisposing risk factor. The following factors have been identified and are generally related to the presence or development of an insulin resistant state:

- breed – donkeys and native ponies are most at risk

- obesity

- pregnancy – increased energy demands particularly in the last trimester

- lactation – increased energy demands

- inadequate exercise

- older age

- gender – females have a higher predisposition.

Irrespective of these risk factors, it is usually a specific event that acts as a trigger to tip the donkey into a negative energy balance, which activates the lipolysis pathway. Hyperlipaemia can be described as either primary or secondary depending on whether the trigger factor is the presence of concurrent disease (secondary) or is related to some other stressor (primary), including:

- excessive/extreme dieting

- management changes

- transport

- loss of a companion

- stress/anxiety

- cereal feeding

- anorexia/reduced appetite
- unexplained weight loss.

In many cases where donkeys are anorexic or losing weight there will be an underlying disease process resulting in secondary hyperlipaemia. In a recent study 72% of donkeys presenting with hyperlipaemia had a concurrent disease (Burden *et al*, 2011). The presence of disease rather than the specific disease process appears to be the trigger factor, which could be due to a combination of anorexia/reduced appetite, exacerbation of insulin resistance, and presence of inflammatory mediators. The presence of dental disease has been found to be a risk factor in itself.

Clinical examination

Because a negative energy balance is key to the development of hyperlipaemia, information about appetite should be obtained from the owner as well as being observed as part of the examination.

> ⚠ **ALERT**
>
> Donkeys will 'sham' eat when unwell, giving the impression of prehension, mastication and swallowing while actually ingesting very little.

The digestible energy content of the diet of pregnant and lactating female donkeys should also be examined to ensure it is sufficient to meet their increased energy demands. The general suitability of the diet and bedding should also be assessed, because paper bedding and cereal feeding were found to be risk factors for hyperlipaemia. It is also important to identify any other stressors that may have occurred in the preceding few weeks, because there is often a delay between the trigger factor and manifestation of clinical signs. Clinical signs are often non-specific and may be related to the primary disease process.

Signs that are often present include:

- dullness
- anorexia/reduced appetite
- reduced gut motility/ileus
- reduced faecal output – dry, mucous covered faeces
- halitosis.

A full clinical examination should be carried out to identify any primary disease process, including a rectal examination both to assess faecal output and to identify any gastrointestinal abnormalities. Studies have reported that 18% of colic cases had secondary hyperlipaemia (Duffield *et al*, 2002).

➲ *See Appendix 1 for a summary of the clinical examination.*

In view of the potential sequelae of pancreatitis, signs of endotoxaemia should also be assessed. The Donkey Sanctuary have found that the most common concurrent diseases have been reported as colic, respiratory disease, laminitis and renal disease.

Diagnosis

Clinical suspicion of hyperlipaemia should be evident from the presentation of an inappetent and/or sick donkey. However, due to the non-specific nature of clinical signs, a blood sample to measure serum triglycerides is required to confirm the diagnosis.

- Take blood early during the examination. Grossly cloudy serum or plasma may be obvious, which enables prompt treatment prior to knowing an exact value for triglycerides.

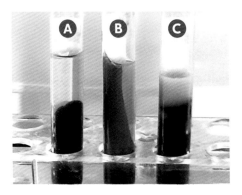

Clotted blood samples showing (A) normal clear serum, (B) slightly cloudy serum where triglycerides will be moderately elevated and (C) milky white serum where the triglycerides will be severely elevated. Note that clear serum does not rule out mild hyperlipaemia.

- The Donkey Sanctuary's normal range for serum triglycerides is 0.6– 2.8 mmol/l (53.4–249.2 mg/dl).

- Liver parameters are also likely to be elevated although it can be difficult to determine whether this is cause or effect because high circulating levels of triglycerides can lead to the development of fatty liver.

- Other biochemical and/or haematological abnormalities may give an indication of the primary disease process or the development of pancreatitis.

Treatment

The restoration of a positive energy balance is of utmost importance in the treatment of hyperlipaemia. In addition, it is vital to **identify the instigating cause for the hyperlipaemia** and to treat this promptly.

Restoring positive energy balance

➜ *See Chapter 18: Nutrition for more information.*

The restoration of a positive energy balance will stimulate endogenous insulin secretion and switch off lipolysis.

Exact energy requirements for sick donkeys are not known. However, **reversal of hyperlipaemia can often be achieved with 60—70kJ/kg bwt/ day** even though this is lower than maintenance requirements.

As guidance:

- In mild cases, support may be given by dosing or in-feed glucose at 1-2g/kg bwt 2 to 3 times a day.

- Enteral feeding may be sufficient where triglycerides are modestly increased (less than 10 mmol/l) and there is some evidence of voluntary food intake and an absence of major secondary disease.

> ⚠ **ALERT**
>
> A ground oat breakfast cereal can provide an instant energy boost in a form that can easily be given using a small bore nasogastric tube and is useful to have to hand when visiting a dull or sick donkey.

- Pelleted high-fibre feeds or a ground oat instant breakfast cereal (for example, Ready Brek 1.5 MJ/100g) can be mixed with water, electrolytes and glucose and administered 2 to 3 times a day through a small bore nasogastric tube. Pre- and probiotics can also be added.

> ⓘ **INFORMATION**
>
> **Example feed to restore a positive energy balance in the donkey**
>
> Administer using a pony or foal size nasogastric tube
>
> - 2-3L warm water (approx 1L / 75kg body weight)
>
> - Rehydration salts (e.g. Effydral™ or Lectade™)
>
> - 120g glucose powder (note that Lectade™ contains approx 50g glucose)
>
> - 250-500g Ready Brek (add the Ready Brek to the water at the last minute to prevent excessive thickening and blockage of the nasogastric tube. Stir well)
>
> - Add any other oral medication to save drenching later

- Where triglycerides are more markedly elevated; higher than 10 mmol/l, it may be possible to administer bolus of intravenous fluids in the home. Mix:

  - 3L Hartmann's with

  - Dextrose at 1-2ml/kg bwt and

  - Duphalyte (solution of B-vitamins, electrolytes, amino-acids and dextrose) at 1—2ml/kg bwt

- In some cases a combination of enteral feeding and intravenous fluids provides the best outcome.

- In more severe cases, donkeys have the best chance of recovery if hospitalised and administered parenteral nutrition.

Parenteral nutrition should be considered when the donkey does not significantly improve after 48 hours.

The following protocol requires close monitoring it should be undertaken in a hospital, where possible, using and infusion pump and with regular monitoring of glucose levels:

> ℹ️ **INFORMATION**
>
> **Example for parenteral nutrition to restore a positive energy balance in a donkey with severe hyperlipaemia**
>
> - Administer an equal mix of 50% glucose and 15% amino acid (such as Aminoven 25, Fresnius Kabi) intravenously at a rate of 0.5ml/kg bwt/h.
>
> - Measure serum glucose every 4 hours.
>
> - Measure triglycerides every 8 hours; a plasma response is generally expected within 12 hours.

- In the field a less intensive regime may provide sufficient levels to restore normal triglycerides in many of the less severe cases. Use:

  - Hartmann's drip at 60ml/kg/day with

  - 5% dextrose added at 1-2ml/kg and

  - Duphalyte (solution of B-vitamins, electrolytes, amino-acids and dextrose) at 100mls/50kg bwt.

> ⚠️ **ALERT**
>
> Any companion(s) should accompany the patient into hospital in order to limit any additional stress from separation and to encourage appetite.

Maintaining some voluntary food intake improves the prognosis.

Appetite can be stimulated by offering the donkey:

- treats such as chopped apples, grated carrots, bananas (particularly the skin) and mints

- cut brambles or allowing the donkey to browse in hedgerows – this can be effective in mild cases and during the recovery period

- flavour enhancers such as peppermint cordial, dried or fresh mint, ginger and fruit juices such as cherry, apple and carrot.

Pain and anti-inflammatory medication

- Remember that inappetent donkeys are also at risk of gastric ulceration, which can be exacerbated by use of non-steroidal anti-inflammatories, so gastro-protection with a therapeutic dose of omeprazole or other effective agents is recommended.

- Pain will often result in inappetence, so if there is any suspicion that the donkey is in pain ensure that analgesic therapy is sufficient to control any signs of pain, which can be very subtle.

- As inflammatory mediators can stimulate lipolysis and inhibit VLDL clearance, if any inflammatory disease such as enterocolitis or peritonitis is suspected, use of anti-inflammatory medication is recommended at dosing intervals suitable for donkeys.

- In view of the risk of endotoxaemia associated with the development of pancreatitis, **flunixin may be the anti-inflammatory of choice in many cases.**

➡ *See Chapter 17: Pharmacology and Therapeutics for more information.*

Prognosis

Successful treatment is more likely if intervention is rapid and energy supply is restored by enteral and/or parenteral feeding alongside appropriate treatment of any underlying condition.

The Donkey Sanctuary has found a mortality rate of 48.5% with the clinical outcome being dependent on the severity of hyperlipaemia such that the survival rate dropped to 30% in donkeys with triglycerides greater than 15mmol/l. It has also been found that donkeys with normal body condition are more likely to survive while donkeys with concurrent disease were less likely to survive.

PITUITARY PARS INTERMEDIA DYSFUNCTION (PPID)

Pituitary pars intermedia dysfunction (PPID), also known as Cushing's disease, is recognised in donkeys. Hirsutism and curliness of the coat are less frequently seen in the PPID donkey. Clinical symptoms may include:

- high internal and external parasite burdens; individual donkeys with consistently high faecal worm egg counts may be affected by PPID

- poorly healing wounds or recurrent infections

- **recurrent, acute or unrecognised laminitis**

- weight loss and loss of muscle mass

- behaviour and demeanour change; for example, owners may report a donkey 'slowing up' or lacking in energy.

Diagnosis and treatment currently follow the same guidelines as in horses and ponies.

Donkey specific reference ranges for ACTH testing have been set by The Donkey Sanctuary and can be found at the start of this chapter.

Supportive care, remedial farriery and pergolide medication are the mainstay of treatment.

Pergolide treatment

Clinicians should begin pergolide treatment based on the same dosages as those given for horses and ponies. But be aware that:

- It is important to ensure accurate weight estimation and dosage.

➡ *See Appendix 2: Donkey Weight Estimator for more information.*

- Pergolide may not be licensed or authorised for use in donkeys. Advise owners and follow appropriate legislation.

Pergolide can be associated with anorexia and secondary hyperlipaemia Donkeys must be monitored closely, particularly when commencing treatment.

⚠ **ALERT**

Treatment with pergolide carries a risk of anorexia and secondary hyperlipaemia.

Monitoring the response to treatment and adjusting the pergolide dose should be undertaken as in horses and ponies.

EQUINE METABOLIC SYNDROME (EMS)

Donkeys are potentially more insulin resistant than horses and ponies and obesity is common in many companion donkeys. Therefore EMS should be considered by clinicians.

Recurrent or acute laminitis in an overweight donkey may be indicative of EMS. Clinicians should be aware that fat deposits may be localised, for example to the neck and rump, particularly in older donkeys.

As in horses and ponies, dynamic challenge tests may be of most diagnostic value, particularly if a basal insulin result is equivocal. Adiponectin testing in donkeys is currently under research.

Complete starving of donkeys prior to blood sampling risks inducing hyperlipaemia. At The Donkey Sanctuary donkeys are not starved completely, but are left with access to straw overnight.

Donkey specific reference ranges for insulin testing have been set by The Donkey Sanctuary and can be found at the start of this chapter.

Treatment follows the same guidelines as for horses and ponies. An overweight donkey should have a carefully managed diet programme to facilitate appropriate weight loss without risking hyperlipaemia.

➡ *See Chapter 18: Nutrition for more information.*

Exercising the donkey can present challenges as EMS-afflicted animals often lead a sedentary existence. Once the clinician is satisfied that any episodes of laminitis are under control, the owner should be encouraged to exercise the donkey. Gentle walking in hand and regular turn out onto bare pasture is appropriate.

Medication may be used in challenging cases, where diet change and exercise combined with appropriate weight loss alone have been ineffective.

Laminitis may be the only indicator that a donkey is affected by PPID or EMS. The clinician should take time to carefully examine the feet and radiograph if there is any doubt. It is essential to provide appropriate analgesia and hoof support if a donkey is affected with laminitis.

➡ *See Chapter 9: The Musculoskeletal Chapter for more information.*

PREVENTION

Be aware of and, where possible, avoid the risk factors and potential stresses associated with hyperlipaemia:

- Maintain a fit and healthy body condition score (Donkey BCS 2.5 -3).

➔ *See Chapter 18: Nutrition for more information.*

- Apply an appropriate preventative health programme including dental care, parasite control, regular foot care and vaccination.

- Ensure appropriate exercise is encouraged, even in older donkeys, either by walking in hand or through creative use of moveable fencing.

🐴 MULES AND HINNIES

There is limited information or evidence available for endocrine disorders in mules and therefore nothing to add that is specific to the mule.

ℹ️ FURTHER INFORMATION

Factsheets, research and detailed information can be found online at: **thedonkeysanctuary.org.uk/for-professionals**

Burden, F.A., Du Toit, N., Hazell-Smith, E. and Trawford, A.F. (2011) Hyperlipemia in a population of aged donkeys: description, prevalence and potential risk factors. *J Vet Intern Med* 25: 1420—1425.

Reid, S.W.J. and Cowan, S.J. (1995) Risk factors for hyperlipaemia in the donkey. *Equine Vet Educ* 7(1): 22—24.

Burden, F.A., Hazell-Smith, E., Mulugeta, G., Patrick, V., Trawford, R. and Brooks Brownlie, H.W. (2016) Reference intervals for biochemical and haematological parameters in mature domestic donkeys (*Equus asinus*) in the UK. *Equine Vet Educ* 28(3): 134—139.

Durham, A.E. and Thiemann, A.K. (2015) Nutritional management of hyperlipaemia. *Equine Vet Educ* 27(9): 482—488.

Burden, F.A. (2012) Practical feeding and condition scoring for donkeys. *Equine Vet Educ* 24(11): 589—596.

Durham, A.E. (2006) Clinical application of parenteral nutrition in the treatment of five ponies and one donkey with hyperlipaemia. *Vet Rec* 158: 159—164.

8. THE SKIN

While the majority of skin conditions seen in donkeys are similar to those found in horses and ponies, there are some characteristics and skin adaptations in the donkey that need to be considered.

Skin conditions tend to be in the advanced stages before they are presented because a thorough examination of the donkey is rarely carried out on a regular basis and the thick coat may hide early problems. Conditions in working donkeys tend to be caused by tack-related issues such as pressure sores due to ill-fitting harnesses or bits.

Poor detection of skin disease is exacerbated by the donkey's stoic nature and reluctance to display signs of discomfort until lesions are advanced.

CLINICAL EXAMINATION

INFECTIOUS DISEASES

PARASITIC DISEASES

OTHER CONDITIONS

WOUNDS

PREVENTION

KEY POINTS

- Donkeys in temperate climates tend to be affected by skin conditions that may be related to the weather conditions and particularly wet weather and lack of shelter.

- Working donkeys tend to suffer from tack-related conditions such as pressure sores.

- It is easy to miss infestation with ectoparasites because of the long coat.

- Many donkeys are not protected by vaccination against tetanus. Check tetanus protection and consider tetanus prophylaxis for all deep wounds, especially of the hoof.

PREVENTION

- Groom donkeys on a daily basis and undertake a thorough whole body check for skin disease and neoplasia in order to allow early detection.

The donkey typically has a long and dry coat and it is often difficult to see ectoparasites such as lice and ticks. Wounds may be missed and skin disease may be in the advanced stages before it is visible.

The long coat is also an important factor to consider when applying topical treatments as dispersal may not be as effective as in horses and ponies and the donkey may not respond to the drug. Drugs applied as a pour-on may not be effective in the donkey.

The donkey has evolved to live in an arid climate and its coat and skin have adapted to this environment.

⚠ **ALERT**

Shelter is essential for the donkey and skin conditions may occur as a result of a lack of shelter in wet weather.

Wet weather can cause problems for donkeys and they will always seek shelter in wet or cold weather. If shelter is not available to them, skin conditions may result. Rugs may be used in addition to shelter and may also be used in cold weather. The Donkey Sanctuary advises the use of donkey shaped rugs.

 *See online at **thedonkeysanctuary.org.uk/for-professionals** for more information on donkey shaped rugs.*

The large ears of the donkey can result in significant heat loss in temperate climates, and prolonged wetting can predispose them to dermatophilus. They can also be an obvious site for sarcoid development and fungal lesions.

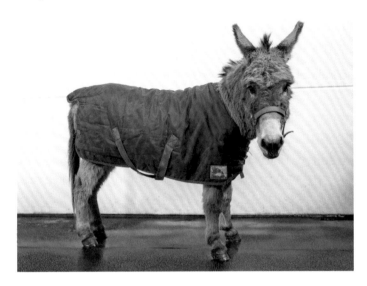

Rugs designed specifically for the donkey are shaped to allow the legs to move freely.

CLINICAL EXAMINATION

➡ *See Appendix 1 for a summary of the clinical examination.*

The following points are important to consider when examining for conditions of the skin:

- Palpate all areas as the longer coat can hide lesions, lumps and parasites.

- Assess the body condition score to check the long coat is not hiding weight loss.

- Skin disease presenting alongside weight loss may signify a systemic aetiology.

- A full blood profile and ACTH testing is recommended in challenging cases and it is important to remember that liver pathology may give rise to clinical signs of skin disease.

- The skin and coat changes apparent in the horse and pony as a result of Pituitary pars intermedia dysfunction (PPID) may be less apparent in the donkey. This may be due to the different management practices for donkeys, for example they are often not groomed regularly.

➡ *See Chapter 7: Hyperlipaemia and the Endocrine System for more information.*

- Clip away the hair from any identified lesion, so that the full extent and character of the lesion can be determined.

- If a tumour is identified, establish the size and characteristics. Check the whole animal as more than one lesion may be present.

- Observe and map the affected areas as this can be very useful for assessing progress and for follow up.

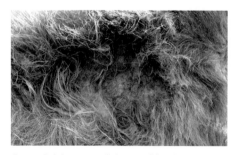 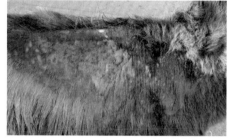

Superficial areas of dermatitis obscured initially by long, matted hair.

Full extent of dermatitis revealed once the hair is clipped away.

Relevant questions for the clinical history would include:

- Are the donkey's companions or handlers affected?

- Have there been any changes to feed or environment?

- Is there a previous history of skin disease and is it seasonal?

- Are there any concerns over the systemic health of the donkey?

- Has there been a history of ectoparasite infestation?

- What is the nutritional status? Donkey diets may be deficient in vitamins and minerals, which can compromise skin health.

➜ *See Chapter 18: Nutrition for more information.*

- Are there any environmental factors such as low lying water and wooded areas providing a suitable habitat for biting insects?

INFECTIOUS SKIN DISEASE

Dermatophytosis (ringworm) is diagnosed and treated as in horses and ponies; although the lesions may be much less obvious. Small alopecic patches may be the only sign. Widespread alopecia with crusting and excoriation may be present.

Remember the zoonotic implications of ringworm.

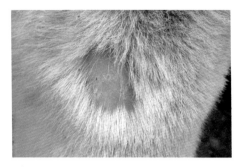

Ringworm on the muzzle of a donkey.

Histoplasmosis (Epizootic lymphangitis) and **Cryptococcosis** are found in donkeys. They are diagnosed and treated as in horses and ponies.

Bacterial infections are usually secondary. They are diagnosed and treated as in horses and ponies.

Viral infections are found in the donkey. They are diagnosed and treated as in horses and ponies.

PARASITIC DISEASE

The donkey is affected by the same parasitic diseases as horses and ponies and are diagnosed and treated similarly.

➡ *See Chapter 11: Parasitology for more information.*

Pediculosis is common in temperate climates. The long coat of the donkey will often hide the presence of lice until there is a heavy infestation. However, clinical presentation varies with individuals: some donkeys are seemingly unaffected by heavy burdens while small burdens result in intense self-trauma in others.

The treatment of lice infestation in the donkey is more successful if any long coat is clipped; allowing effective dispersal of topical treatment and better visibility of the site. Clipping can also increase UV exposure to the skin, which can be helpful.

It may be necessary to apply larger volumes of licensed topical preparations due to the coat differences. It is important to note that a resistance has been identified in some of the preparations licensed for equines.

It is worth establishing the type of louse present in a case before selecting treatment as this may determine whether topical or systemic treatment is appropriate.

Amongst the UK Donkey Sanctuary herd the chewing louse, *Bovicola (Werneckiella) ocellatus* is prevalent and has been shown to be resistant to topical permethrins. However in other donkey populations where chewing lice are present it may be appropriate to consider the use of topical permethrin.

(Systemic avermectin may be used where sucking lice have been identified).

Topical application of fipronil has also proved efficacious in the treatment of lice infestations but clinicians must remember that larger volumes may be required to penetrate the donkey's thick coat if clipping is not performed.

The use of a topical 5% tea tree oil product has been shown to be an alternative option to permethrin based compounds. One option is 'Equine Nit Nat' which was developed with The Donkey Sanctuary.

➡ *See online at* **agrientlimited.com/equine-nitnat** *for more information on 'Equine Nit Nat'.*

⚠ **ALERT**

The long thick coat of the donkey will affect topical application of drugs. Larger volumes or clipping may be necessary.

Flies and Midges (*Culicoides spp*) will have the same effect on donkeys as in horses and ponies. They are prone to fly bite attacks, predominantly on the distal limbs and in elderly and arthritic donkeys who are less mobile. Hypersensitivity to fly bites or to Culicoides bites (Sweet Itch) will result in pruritic papules and nodule formation.

Flies can act as vectors for other disease such as habronemiasis.

Prevention of fly attack relies on good hygiene and environmental measures in the same way as is recognised for horses and ponies.

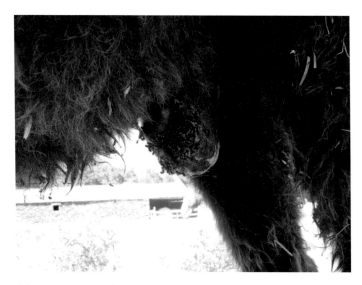

The sheath of a donkey can be prone to fly attack and can become affected with habronemiasis as a result.

Pinworm *Oxyuris equi* infestation can be easily mistaken for Culicoides bites in donkeys. It frequently presents with hair breakage and excoriation of the rump, tail head and perianal region.

Mites infest donkeys in the same way as horses and ponies. Forage mites and *Chorioptes spp* may be seen and, rarely, the burrowing mites, *Sarcoptes spp* and *Demodex spp*. Donkeys fed and bedded on straw may have an increased likelihood of infestation with forage mites due to an increased exposure. They are often found around the head for this reason.

Ticks present problems as they are very difficult to find in the donkey coat. Donkeys are susceptible to tick-borne infections as in horses and ponies.

Habronemiasis and Onchocerciasis are found in donkeys. They are diagnosed and treated as in horses and ponies.

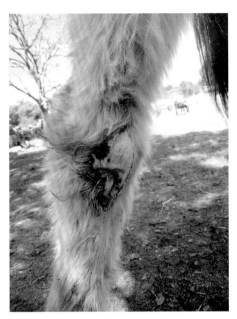 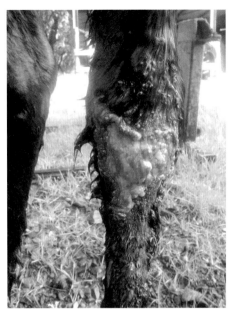

Severe habronemiasis affecting the limb of a donkey.

Ivermectin can be mixed with vaseline and used topically for habronemiasis in areas of the donkey that are problematic for treatment, such as the skin around the eye and the sheath. This will also protect the wound against flies during the period of treatment.

➔ *See online at **thebrooke.org/for-professionals/working-equid-veterinary-manual** for more information in The Working Equid Veterinary Manual.*

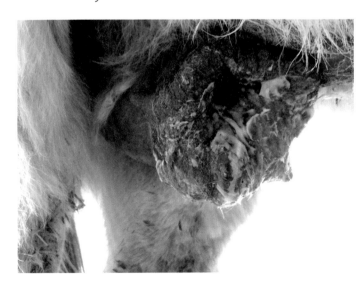

Application of ivermectin mixed with Vaseline on the sheath of a donkey affected with habronemiasis.

OTHER CONDITIONS

Sarcoids have been identified in the donkey and are presented as in horses and ponies.

Treatment is the same as in horses and ponies and it is important to note that:

- Early recognition and prompt treatment of a sarcoid facilitates the chance of successful therapy. Donkeys should be checked regularly, particularly the sheath and inguinal areas.

- Surgical or chemotherapeutic intervention, as in horses and ponies, remains the mainstay of therapy and laser or smart surgery with wide local margins are currently the most successful approaches. Multimodal therapy using surgery and adjunctive chemo or radiotherapy may be required.

- Specialist opinion should always be sought if there is any doubt over a treatment plan.

- Recurrence rates are high and owners and vets should be ever vigilant.

Other neoplastic diseases have been seen and should be considered as part of the differential diagnosis:

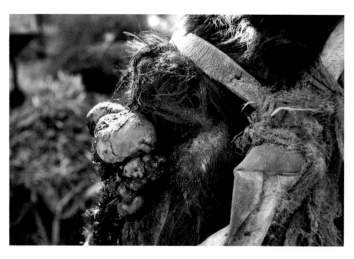

Aggressive fibroblastic sarcoid.

Melanoma appears to have a low incidence despite the high numbers of donkeys with a grey coloured coat.

Squamous Cell Carcinoma has been recorded in cutaneous, ocular and genital forms and should be investigated and treated as in horses and ponies.

Fibromas/fibrosarcoma have occasionally been diagnosed by histopathology in suspected sarcoid lesions. However, several authors consider these to be variants of the sarcoid and manage them as such.

Insect bite hypersensitivity is found in donkeys but it can be difficult to distinguish between hypersensitivity to the bite of *Culicoides spp* or to fly-bites. Hypersensitivity is diagnosed and treated as in horses and ponies.

Atopic dermatitis presents and is treated in the same way as in horse and ponies.

Vasculitis is rare in the donkey but when seen it should be treated in the same way as in horses and ponies.

Autoimmune diseases have been recorded in the donkey, *Pemphigus foliaceous* being the most relevant. The prognosis is guarded.

Congenital diseases are rare in the donkey but junctional epidermal bullosa has been recorded.

Besnoitiosis may be seen as donkeys appear susceptible to the protozoal parasite *Besnoitia bennetti.*

Molluscum contagiosum, the pox virus, has recently been described in two donkeys.

WOUNDS

Approaches to the treatment and prevention of skin wounds in donkeys is the same as in horses and ponies.

Remember that donkeys may not be protected against tetanus and appropriate prophylactic treatment must be given.

Wounds may be advanced and possibly secondarily infected as the long coat of the donkey may hide wounds, and any grooming or examinations are often undertaken infrequently.

In working donkeys repetitive trauma arising from poor tack, carrying of inappropriate loads, and debilitated donkeys suffering from poor nutrition, can lead to severe wounds. In these cases the cause of the wound has to be addressed in order to prevent re-occurrence. This may involve education and advice on alternative options for the owner or the community.

 See online at **thedonkeysanctuary.org.uk/for-professionals** *for more information in The Good Harness Guide.*

⚠ ALERT

Many donkeys are not vaccinated against tetanus and prophylactic treatment may be necessary.

PREVENTION

The prevention of skin wounds is an important consideration. Owners should be advised to:

- Vaccinate against tetanus.

- Undertake regular and thorough examination of the coat combined with daily grooming.

- Seek expert advice as soon as a problem is identified.

- Use correct and well-fitted equipment, especially harnesses and bits.

- Adapt tack to allow for any skin conditions or musculo-skeletal conditions, to minimise pressure sores or rubbing.

- Change or adapt management and working practices that contribute to the development of wounds.

*See online at **thebrooke.org/for-professionals/working-equid-veterinary-manual** for more information on wound control in The Working Equid Veterinary Manual.*

🐴 MULES AND HINNIES

- The less dense coat of many mules facilitates visual assessment.

- The temperament of the mule may hinder safe close examination.

There is a lack of information or evidence available for skin diseases in mules and therefore nothing to add that is specific to the mule.

ℹ️ FURTHER INFORMATION

Factsheets, research and detailed information can be found online at: **thedonkeysanctuary.org.uk/for-professionals**

The Good Harness Guide: **thedonkeysanctuary.org.uk/for-professionals**

The Working Equid Veterinary Manual: **thebrooke.org/for-professionals/ working-equid-veterinary-manual**

Ellse, L., Burden, F. and Wall, R. (2012) Pyrethroid tolerance in the chewing louse *Bovicola (Werneckiella) ocellatus. Veterinary Parasitology.*

Ellse, L., Sands, B., Burden, F.A. and Wall, R. (2016) Essential oils in the management of the donkey louse *Bovicola ocellatus. Equine Veterinary Journal 48* (3), pp 285—289.

Fox, R., Thiemann, A., Everest, D., Steinbach, F., Dastjerdi, A., Finnegan, C. (2012) Molluscum contagiosum in two donkeys. *Veterinary Record* 170 (25), pp 649—651.

Taylor, S. and Haldorson, G. (2013) A Review of Equine Sarcoid. *Equine Veterinary Education* 25 (4) 210—216.

White, S. (2013) Donkey Dermatology. *Veterinary Clinics of North America* 29 (3), pp 703—708.

9. THE MUSCULOSKELETAL SYSTEM

The anatomy and treatment of the musculoskeletal system in donkeys is largely the same as in horses and ponies, with the exception of the foot and it is important to be aware of the differences in the anatomy of the foot, and the associated requirement for different management of conditions.

Conditions of the musculoskeletal system are one of the main reasons for euthanasia, and a lack of regular footcare frequently contributes to this. The stoical nature of the donkey can make lameness diagnosis challenging. This is exacerbated in the companion donkey by a lack of physical exercise, regular inspection and opportunities to be aware of issues.

Laminitis, one of the most common causes of lameness, can easily be overlooked and may go undiagnosed for a considerable time.

Hoof disorders and distal limb osteoarthritis and injury are commonly found in working donkeys globally, where as higher limb joint osteoarthritis is more commonly in older companion animals.

THE NORMAL FOOT

CLINICAL EXAMINATION

COMMON CONDITIONS

PREVENTION

KEY POINTS

- Inadequate footcare and poor farriery are significant welfare issues globally.

- Cases of both acute and chronic lamintis frequently go unrecognised.

- EMS and PPID are important factors in many cases of recurrent and chronic lamintis.

- Humid and muddy environments often predispose to serious foot disease.

- Pus tracking under the hoof wall is a frequent cause of acute severe lameness.

- When assessing lateromedial foot xrays specific donkey data should be used.

The flat withers and back make it more suitable as a pack animal. The stoic nature and stamina of the donkey can lead to overuse, overloading and general abuse that can result in back wounds.

The donkey has some differences in conformation compared to the horse and pony:

- The pectoral muscles are relatively underdeveloped and are not suitable to be used as an injection site.

- The donkey has five lumbar vertebrae.

- The 1st coccygeal vertebrae is often fused to the sacrum, with occlusion of the sacro-coccygeal space.

- The first inter-coccygeal space is narrower than the second, so the preferred injection site for epidural anaesthesia is between C2 and C3.

➔ *See Chapter 15: Euthanasia and the Post-Mortem Examination for more information on anatomy.*

The donkey's foot has several significant anatomical differences to that of the horse and pony:

- a more upright hoof pastern axis

- a dorsal hoof wall that is 5 to 10 degrees more upright

- a broader frog with an apex that does not extend as far towards the toe

- a U-shaped sole slightly flared at the heels

- narrower heels resulting in a cylindrical shaped hoof capsule

- a thicker sole

- a constant hoof-wall thickness from heel to toe

- the extensor process of the distal phalanx is located distal to the upper limit of the hoof capsule in normal feet; lateral radiographs should be interpreted accordingly

- microscopically, horn tubule size, density and distribution patterns differ from those of the horse.

Studies on donkeys kept in the UK indicate that moisture content of the hoof wall, a major factor in determining its mechanical properties, is significantly higher in donkeys than in horses and ponies, making it more pliant and deformable. This may predispose to hoof capsule disorders and pathological conditions when animals are kept in higher humidity environments.

The donkey foot has a distinctive five-point loading pattern with focal stresses acting at the dorsal aspect of the hoof, the quarters, and the heels, in contrast to the four-point pattern reported in the horse and pony.

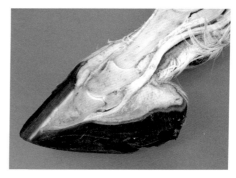

Split section of a donkey hoof showing the position of P3 with relation to the coronary band, and the position of the frog caudally on P3. Note how this makes placing a frog support only on a laminitic donkey foot inappropriate.

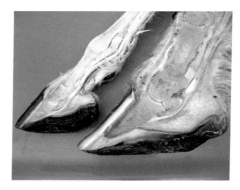

Comparison with the horse and donkey foot.

THE NORMAL FOOT

Depending on the environment and lifestyle, a donkey's feet will generally require trimming every six to ten weeks. Even where donkeys are walking on surfaces that naturally abrade hoof growth, it is recommended that this regular check and trim is not ignored.

Trimming

The limbs should be kept low when trimming and should not be abducted from the body. This will reduce the risk of unbalancing the donkey or causing pain and discomfort in animals that are affected with arthritis. It will also facilitate compliance.

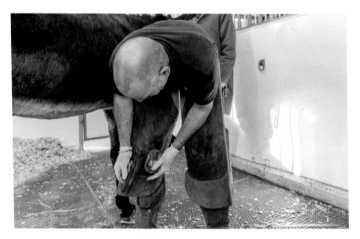

The foot held low for trimming.

When trimming it is important to note the specific differences for the donkey:

- Pare the sole first, removing all loose and necrotic material and paring back any overgrown frog. The frog frequently becomes large and bulbous, with the grooves and sulci retaining foreign matter and infection. The frog should be trimmed to a neat triangular shape, removing all degenerate and overgrown tissue.

- The sole of the donkey does not tend to flake away naturally, unlike the sole of the horse and pony. Consequently it frequently requires paring back so that it ideally becomes concave, minimising the area of sole that will be in contact with the ground and enabling the walls to bear weight. The sole is pared back in increments until thumb pressure between the apex of the frog and the toe causes the sole to yield perceptibly.

- Trim the wall guided by the pastern axis and the angle of the wall at the proximal midline. A straight hoof pastern axis is ideal, with heel height frequently requiring reduction. The well-developed coronary band in some donkeys can be deceptive when assessing the hoof pastern axis. Excessive rasping of the hoof wall should be avoided.

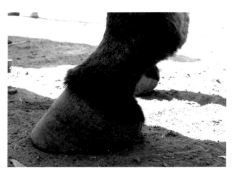 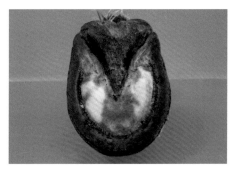

A correctly trimmed donkey hoof.

- Assess the medio-lateral balance as in the horse and pony, and make adjustments so that the weight is transmitted equally across the width of the foot.

- Assess the balance, gait and comfort of the donkey post-trimming.

➜ *See online at* **thedonkeysanctuary.org.uk/for-professionals** *for a video demonstrating trimming of the foot.*

Shoeing

For most activities and in most situations donkeys do not need to be fitted with shoes. When wear is excessive and shoes are required, greater care is needed when placing nails in the narrow upright walls of the donkey hoof.

Many traditional donkey shoes limit or prevent heel expansion. These are not recommended as they restrict the natural functioning of the hoof and may predispose to longer term problems such as atrophy of the frog and broken forward hoof pastern axes.

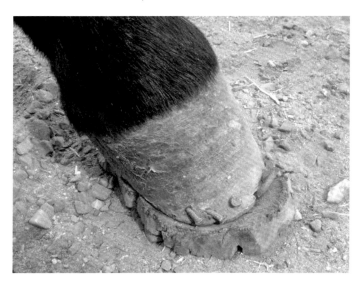

Shoeing a donkey with car tyre rubber shoe and carpentry nails in Mali.

Synthetic shoes that cover the entire solar surface predispose to degeneration and disease of the sole and frog. These should also be avoided.

In cases where it is necessary to relieve sole pressure (eg cases of chronic laminitis), or where rebuilding the hoof wall after remedial farriery or surgery, hoof resins and thermoplastic granule products have proven useful. They are used in the same way as with horses and ponies; ensure that feet are clean and dry for the products to work effectively, and apply in thin layers to avoid tissue damage due to the heat generated when the products harden.

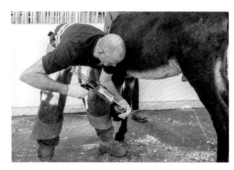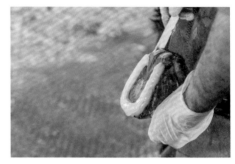

Applying a rim shoe.

CLINICAL EXAMINATION

Donkeys experiencing pain tend to stand still or lie down, hence identification of any lameness or the presence of pain may be difficult and is often delayed.

Hyperlipaemia may occur in association with problems that cause lameness. A full clinical examination is therefore strongly recommended when clinicians are presented with a lame donkey.

It can be challenging to examine for lameness in donkeys because they rarely trot or move at speed when led. In many cases the only way of assessing a donkey's gait is to spend time observing its movements in its natural environment.

Owners may report subtle changes in behaviour, including reduced activity or increasing periods of time spent laying down.

> ⚠ **ALERT**
>
> Response to hoof testers has to be interpreted with caution in donkeys.

Hoof testers may be useful in localising or identifying foot pain, although the results should be interpreted with caution in these stoic animals.

Foot trimming may aid effective examination of the foot.

During feet examinations keep hooves close to the ground to minimise stress on the joints and reduce discomfort to older or arthritic donkeys.

As with horses and ponies, assessing digital pulse intensity is a key part of a lameness examination in the donkey.

Radiography

It is important to note that there are certain key differences in the donkey's foot compared to that of a horse or pony:

- A limited broken forward hoof pastern axis can be considered normal, with a degree of rotation of the dorsal aspect of the distal phalanx in relation to the long axis of the proximal phalanx.

- The distal phalanx is positioned more distally in the hoof capsule resulting in a greater distance between the proximal limit of the hoof wall and the extensor process of the distal phalanx ('founder distance'). The mean founder distance in the standard donkey is reported as 10.4mm (SD +/- 3.66).

- The mean integument depth measured at the midpoint of the distal phalanx is 25% greater in the donkey (16.2mm) than reported in the pony.

The donkey foot displays a parallel relationship between the dorsal hoof wall and the dorsal border of the distal phalanx, in the same way as the horse and pony, in ideal situations. However, this is not always the case, especially in donkeys where regular foot care is neglected.

The angle of the solar surface to the ground is similar to that reported for the horse and pony.

Ultrasonography

Ultrasound examination of the donkey's limbs is undertaken as in horses and ponies. Extra care should be taken to prepare the site prior to ultrasonography in order to ensure good image quality because many donkeys have a thick coat.

COMMON CONDITIONS

The overgrown hoof

Overgrown hooves, with or without twisting, is a common problem in donkeys. In extreme cases hooves can resemble Turkish slippers. However, many less pronounced cases of overgrowth, with painful stress on joints and ligaments, are all too frequently seen.

Lateral radiographs will aid trimming and allow an accurate position of the distal phalanx (P3) to be established and an assessment of any laminitic change to be made. In the absence of radiographs, successful trimming can be undertaken if the position of P3 is estimated from its relationship to the coronary band, bearing in mind that the proximal extensor process will be distal to the coronary band. This distance may be greater in cases of chronic laminitis, a common problem associated with overgrowth.

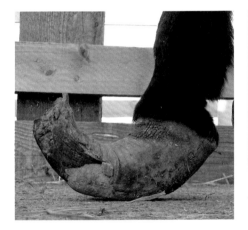 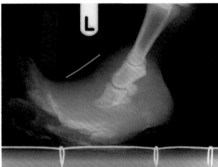

An overgrown hoof and radiograph.

Recommendations for correction are:

- Remove the frog and sole overgrowth and reduce the heels first, in order to allow the bearing surface to sit correctly on the ground,

- remove toe overgrowth. Stop paring when thumb pressure on the sole reveals slight 'give',

- dress back the dorsal wall of the hoof with a rasp once the toe has been removed, guided by the angle of the proximal hoof wall adjacent to the mid coronary band,

- remove degenerate hoof wall and white line if enough wall remains to allow the donkey to move reasonably comfortably.

Pay careful attention to post trimming analgesia. A comfortable, deeply bedded stable, good hoof hygiene, regular inspection, and an appropriate farriery plan for the future should all be considered.

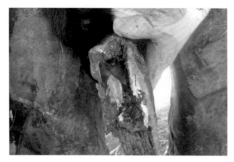

The first stage in trimming this overlong hoof is to trim the heels to a normal angle; the frog is then redefined and the sole is scalloped out gently.

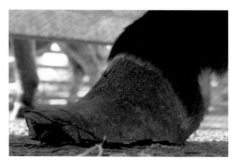

The hoof on the ground showing the heels achieving a more normal relationship with the ground.

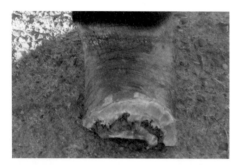

The hoof from the front shows the extent of hoof wall separation due to stretching of the laminae.

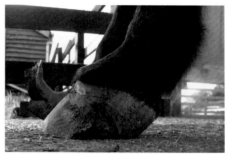

The left fore is nearly finished after one trim; the right has yet to be done. In uncomplicated cases, the hoof can be corrected by a skilful farrier with one trim. Some donkeys may require mild analgesia for a few days after trimming.

Laminitis

This is one of the most common causes of lameness in non-working donkeys. It is often undetected until the condition is advanced. This is possibly due to the stoic nature and non-athletic lifestyle of many donkeys, and the subtlety of a donkey's changes in behaviour in response to pain.

Donkeys with laminitis:

- are reluctant to move
- show a short stride
- are recumbent for more time than usual
- are likely to show signs of weight shifting when on hard ground
- are less likely to show the classical equine laminitic stance unless severely affected.

Examination will identify:

- increased digital pulses

- solar pain that may be localised to an area corresponding to the tip of the distal phalanx

- distortion of the hoof capsule in chronic cases, possibly along with developing muscle wastage around the shoulders, increasing their prominence.

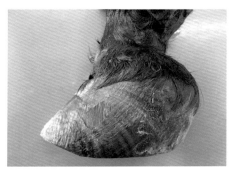

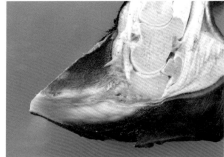

External appearance of donkey hoof with chronic laminitis. Note the obvious laminitic rings that widen towards the heel.

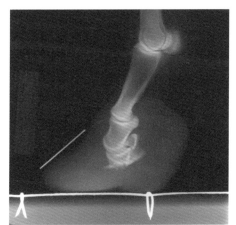

Split section of the hoof, showing severe degeneration of P3 and movement of P3 distally within the hoof capsule.

Lateral radiograph of the hoof, showing tremendous degeneration and distortion of P3.

⚠ **ALERT**

Ranges for the radiographic parameters of the foot differ in donkeys to those of horses and ponies.

Diagnosis will be made on clinical signs and radiographic changes, taking into account the different parameters for normal donkeys. In view of the founder distance in normal donkeys it can be difficult to assess any depression around the coronary band. However, if there is pain associated with this, then it is a significant finding.

Radiographic changes in the laminitic foot of the adult donkey (Collins *et al*, 2011):

Parameter	Normal donkey	Laminitic donkey
	Mean (+/- s.d.)	mean (+/- s.d.)
Founder distance (mm)	10.40 (3.66)	13.02 (3.98)
Angle of solar aspect of DP (degrees)	8.26 (4.75)	10.89 (6.37)
Angle of deviation between dorsal aspect of DP and dorsal hoof wall (degrees)	2.50 (3.07)	12.52 (9.40)
Phalangeal rotation angle (degrees)	-9.39 (9.16)	-14.80 (10.7)
Distal inter-phalangeal rotational angle (degrees)	-4.30 (10.40)	-2.40 (11.60)
Mean integument depth at mid point of DP (mm)	15.60 (2.60)	20.36 (4.13)

(DP = Distal Phalanx)

The aetiology of laminitis in donkeys is similar to that in the horse and pony.

Equine Metabolic Syndrome (EMS) and pituitary pars intermedia dysfunction (PPID) become more significant in elderly and obese animals and are increasingly recognised as an important factor in the aetiology of laminitis in the donkey.

➔ *See Chapter 7: Hyperlipaemia and the Endocrine System for reference ranges for insulin and ACTH.*

- **Treatment** for laminitis in donkeys is similar to treatment in the horse and pony.

- **Dietary management** is essential to control weight, although care needs to be taken with weight loss to ensure that it is not excessive, because this may increase the risk of hyperlipaemia.

⚠ **ALERT**

Weight loss should be gradual. Aim for 2—3% of bodyweight monthly and monitor for signs of hyperlipaemia.

➔ *See Chapter 18: Nutrition for more information.*

- **Medical management** of laminitis in the donkey is similar to that in the horse and pony, although the frequency of dosing for most NSAIDs needs to be increased to twice daily due to differences in drug metabolism when compared to horses and ponies.

⚠ **ALERT**

Phenylbutazone and flunixin should be administered twice daily to donkeys.

When an animal is in acute pain, multimodal analgesia can be helpful, using similar doses of paracetamol, opioids and ketamine to those administered to horses and ponies. Fentanyl patches have also been used on donkeys.

➔ *See Chapter 17: Pharmacology and Therapeutics for more information.*

• **Corrective farriery** is important for rebalancing the foot once the acute phase is over.

The frog of the donkey, although often well developed, tends not to extend as far forwards towards the toe. Pedal bone support by frog supports alone is therefore not helpful and possibly contraindicated. A thick cotton pad covering the whole foot, together with deep bedding, can provide support and comfort.

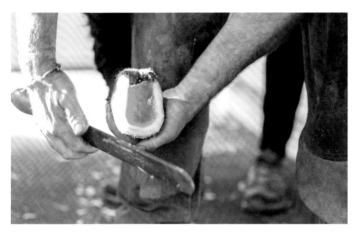

Solar support for the laminitic foot.

⚠ **ALERT**

The use of frog supports is not advisable in the donkey.

Lateromedial radiographs are indicated for assessing prognosis and as an aid to corrective farriery. Interpretation should be carried out using donkey specific ranges shown earlier in this chapter.

Chronic cases can be difficult to assess and radiographs are an essential part of making a diagnosis. Typical changes to the distal phalanx include:

• modelling or lipping of the tip

• demineralisation of the distal margin

• distal displacement within the hoof capsule.

Commercially available therapeutic shoes can be of benefit, although the shape and size of the donkey's hoof can make fitting difficult. The main objective is to remove the load from the sole. Hoof resins can be used to recreate the hoof wall.

After the acute phase, exercise can also be beneficial to control weight and provide enrichment.

White line disease

Donkeys in some environments appear prone to white line disease. Dirty, wet conditions, genetic factors, mechanical stress and poor farriery are cited as causes. Lesions can extend around the circumference of the hoof and progress proximally towards the coronary band.

Donkey hooves have a higher moisture content in certain environments than horse and pony hooves, which may exacerbate the problem. Repeated bouts of laminitis weaken the sole/wall junction, providing an ideal route for keratolytic fungi and bacteria to invade.

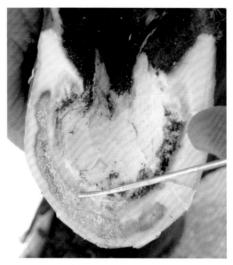

White line disease before debridement.

The condition is characterised by crumbly grey/white material at the sole/wall junction. Donkeys are not usually lame, although in severe cases deep pockets of black, foul-smelling discharge may cause lameness and sensitivity to hoof testers.

Treatment is aimed at debriding all affected horn, rebalancing the foot and providing a dry, clean environment. Donkeys can cope with extensive debridement around the toe, but radiographs are advised where concurrent signs of chronic laminitis and thin soles are seen.

White line abscess

These can be very frustrating to deal with because there is rarely an obvious lesion, and many hooves have stretched white lines and multiple areas of white line disease to explore. It may be possible to localise the abscess if small, lightweight hoof testers are used. However, some larger, thick-soled breeds, such as Poitous, show little response to the hoof tester.

Thorough initial trimming of the hoof is recommended; remove all but the deeper lesions. Difficult cases can benefit from a bilateral abaxial sesamoid nerve block alongside poulticing and hot tubbing, to encourage pus to drain.

Pus may move more dorsally in more longstanding cases, or inwards towards the pedal bone. Pus rarely underruns the sole in donkeys. Radiographs are indicated if pus has not drained and the donkey has been severely lame for more than two days.

Lame donkeys should always be monitored for appetite and signs of hyperlipaemia.

Tetanus prophylaxis must be considered and adequate analgesia provided to maintain comfort and promote appetite.

> ⚠ **ALERT**
>
> In donkeys pus tends to move dorsally under the hoof wall, or towards the pedal bone, rather than under the sole.

Chronic foot disease

Chronic foot disease is a descriptive term used to categorise cases with any or all; chronic laminitis, white line disease, pedal bone degeneration and pain. It may be possible to keep such cases comfortable with the long-term use of NSAIDs, careful farriery, level pastures and soft bedding. It is essential that the quality of life of affected donkeys is regularly assessed, with objective recording of assessments being very useful in helping decide when euthanasia is appropriate.

 See Chapter 14: The Geriatric Donkey for more information on Quality of Life assessments.

These cases respond poorly to stress and the increased weight-bearing associated with transportation. Clinicians should therefore be particularly careful when assessing the fitness to travel of such donkeys.

Keratomas

Keratomata are seen in donkeys, affecting both front and hind feet. Clinical signs include repeat abscess-like lameness with pus frequently discharging at the coronary band. In some cases there is associated deformation of the hoof wall.

Dorso-proxima—palmarodistal oblique radiographs will reveal a smooth defect in the margin of the distal phalanx. Surgical removal is required but recurrence can be an issue.

Distal interphalangeal joint hyperflexion

Due to the naturally upright hoof pastern angle of the donkey, distal interphalangeal joint hyperflexion ('ballerina syndrome') is not always detected early. The condition is usually but not exclusively seen in young, rapidly growing donkeys fed in excess of their requirements. It is also seen in working donkeys in association with foot injury and distal joint arthritis.

In mild cases the heel will be raised but the dorsal wall will not be beyond the vertical. In more severe cases the dorsal hoof wall tips beyond the vertical with a marked reduction in the heel to fetlock distance.

Mild cases may respond to a combination of diet restriction, corrective farriery, extension shoes and analgesia. More severe cases require surgical intervention. Pre-treatment radiography is recommended.

The condition is also seen in geriatric donkeys, where it may be linked to chronic pain in the upper limb.

Angular limb deformities

These are found in donkeys and are treated as in horses and ponies. However, in many cases they are left untreated because the donkey is not going to be an athlete. This may present a problem later in life due to the development of secondary degenerative joint disease (DJD).

At the stage where secondary DJD has developed, the deformity can only be managed with pain relief using NSAIDs.

Osteoarthritis

Osteoarthritis is a common problem in geriatric donkeys and frequently affects the upper limb joints, primarily the shoulders and hips. Signs may be subtle and only noticed when lesions are chronic and severe. These include:

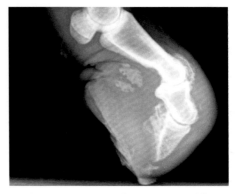

Digital hyperflexion with osteoarthritis that might preclude effective treatment.

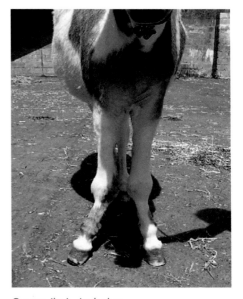

Severe limb deviation.

- shortened stride length

- difficulty getting up or reluctance to lie down

- resentment when having limbs lifted for routine procedures such as foot cleaning or farriery.

Working donkeys may be more likely to show signs of DJD in the lower limb joints. The changes can be chronic and severe, resulting in partial or complete joint fusion.

Ankylosing spondylitis of the cervical, but more often, the thoracic spine can also occur as part of the ageing process.

Treatment of the donkey will be similar to that of the horse and pony, although the frequency of dosing for most NSAIDs needs to be increased to twice daily due to the different drug metabolism of the donkey.

Regular monitoring and assessment of quality of life is recommended.

➡ *See Chapter 17: Pharmacology and Therapeutics for more information on doses.*

Tendonitis/desmitis

Working donkeys in particular frequently suffer from chronic tendonitis and desmitis, caused or exacerbated by trauma, fatigue, abnormal loads and poor farriery.

Presentation and treatment is the same as in horse and ponies.

Stringhalt

Aging donkeys are occasionally seen with a sporadic involuntary flexion of one or both hind limbs. The severity and frequency varies and it is speculatively considered to be similar to stringhalt in horses and ponies. No effective treatment has been identified, but affected donkeys may survive many years untroubled by the condition.

PREVENTION

The prevention of hoof disorders relies on the following throughout the life of the donkey:

- appropriate nutrition and maintenance of a healthy body condition score (2.5 – 3)

- regular foot care and farriery appropriate to the specific needs of the donkey

- a dry, clean environment, including stabling and exercise area

- prompt attention as soon as signs of lameness are seen.

🐾 MULES AND HINNIES

- The internal anatomy of the mule's foot is similar to that of the horse and pony.

- Mules have the same number of lumbar vertebrae as horses and ponies.

- Mules are less prone to white line disease than donkeys.

ℹ️ FURTHER INFORMATION

Factsheets, research and detailed information can be found online at:
thedonkeysanctuary.org.uk/for-professionals

Collins, S.N., Dyson, S.J., Murray, R.C., Burden, F. & Trawford, A. (2011) Radiological anatomy of the donkey's foot: Objective characterisation of the normal and laminitic donkey foot. *Equine Veterinary Journal* 43 (4), 478—486.

Grosenbaugh, D.A., Reinemeyer, C.R. and Figueiredo, M.D. (2011) Pharmacology and therapeutics in donkeys. *Equine Veterinary Education* 23 (10), 523—530.

Thiemann, A.K. and Rickards, K. (2013) Donkey hoof disorders and their treatment. *In Practice* 35, 135—140.

10. INFECTIOUS DISEASES

Specific, validated information on the epidemiology and manifestation of infectious diseases in donkeys and mules is frequently limited or lacking. Donkey specific differences are discussed where they are supported by evidence or experience both in the notifiable infectious diseases, as included in the OIE's (World Organisation for Animal Health) 2018 list of diseases, and in other infectious diseases. Where a disease is not included, reference should be made to general equine texts and information.

Prevention is an important consideration for infectious diseases in any species and revolves around sound biosecurity principles, early detection and vaccination where available.

NOTIFIABLE INFECTIOUS DISEASES

OTHER INFECTIOUS DISEASES

PREVENTION

KEY POINTS

- Donkeys can be affected by those infectious diseases that affect horses and ponies, although the epidemiology and clinical presentation may differ.

- Many diagnostic methodologies used for horses and ponies have not been validated or tested specifically for donkeys.

- Many drugs and vaccines have not been licensed for donkeys.

- It is essential to be aware of the diseases that are zoonotic and to consider public health implications.

- Clinical examination, especially oral examination of donkeys suspected of infection with rabies, requires particular care.

NOTIFIABLE INFECTIOUS DISEASES

The infectious diseases discussed in this section are those included in the OIE's single list of notifiable diseases. The current global status for each disease can be found on the OIE website. This section only includes information that is specific to the donkey.

 *See online at **oie.int/en/animal-health-in-the-world/oie-listed-diseases-2018** for more information.*

Each country will have local regulations for the reporting of these diseases and it is important to be aware of them and of the protocols for notification.

African Horse Sickness (AHS)

The infectious agent is the orbivirus and transmission is by midges.

AHS is usually subclinical but mild clinical signs can be seen in the donkey.

Note that:

- Asian and European donkeys are moderately susceptible, with 5—10% mortality.

- African donkeys, where the disease is endemic, are often described as relatively resistant and considered as reservoir hosts. However, they have been shown to become viraemic following inoculation with virulent AHS virus, and have been seen to exhibit a mild form of the disease, 'horse sickness fever'.

- Where clinical signs are seen, they are typically:

  - high fever

  - weakness

  - dyspnoea

  - extensive oedema of the supraorbital fossae and the eyelids.

- Congestion and haemorrhage of conjunctivae were also observed in donkeys in Kenya, which were serologically positive for AHS virus.

- Mortality of donkeys with typical clinical signs of the pulmonary form of AHS, characterised by dyspnoea and terminal frothy nasal exudate, has been seen in Ethiopia.

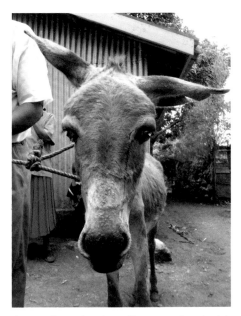

A prominent head swelling associated with oedema of the supraorbital fossae and eyelids, congestion and haemorrhage of the conjunctivae.

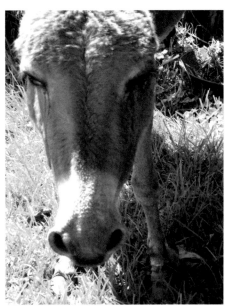

Fully dilated nostrils with extended head and abducted forelegs.

Equine Herpes virus (EHV)

A similar range of herpes virus affect donkeys as those in horses and ponies.

Clinical signs are similar to those seen in horses and ponies.

Infection can be treated as in horses and ponies, but with some differences.

➡ *See chapter 4: The Respiratory System for more information.*

Equine Influenza

Equine Influenza presents with the same clinical signs seen in horses and ponies. However, there are reports that donkeys may be more severely affected.

➡ *See chapter 4: The Respiratory System for more information.*

Equine Infectious Anaemia (EIA)

The infectious agent is the lentivirus and transmission is by biting insects.

EIA is usually subclinical in the donkey.

There is limited information on the epidemiology of EIA in donkeys.

Equine Viral Arteritis (EVA)

The infectious agent is the arterivirus and transmission is via secretions from the respiratory or reproductive systems.

EVA is usually subclinical but mild clinical signs may be seen in the donkey.

Note that:

- There is one major serotype, but different isolates have been recognised in donkeys, mules and horses.

- Studies have demonstrated natural infection in donkeys and they can be clinically affected, although signs are not as severe as in horses and ponies.

- Where **clinical signs** are evident, they are typically:

  - fever

  - depression

  - ocular and nasal discharge

  - conjunctivitis.

- Respiratory and venereal routes of transmission of EVA have been reported in donkeys.

- An asinine virus closely related to the equine arteritis virus has been isolated from donkey semen.

- Affected male donkeys may become long-term carriers and may shed the virus in their semen, serving as reservoirs for the virus.

Rabies

The infectious agent is the lyssavirus and transmission is the bite of an infected animal.

Donkeys typically show the encephalitic and paralytic form.

Note that:

- Working donkeys usually become infected with rabies from the bites of infected carnivores, in particular dogs, jackals, hyenas and foxes.

- Working donkeys are more at risk because they are often kept outside at night or allowed to wander freely.

- Vampire bat-transmitted rabies in donkeys has been reported in Mexico and reports from Latin America suggest that donkeys are more likely than horses and ponies to be attacked by vampire bats.

- **Donkeys may show vague, non-specific signs, such as depression, anorexia, apparent choke (oesophageal obstruction) and colic at the early stages of the disease.**

- **'Furious' (neurological) signs are common in the advanced stage of the disease and are characterised by aggressive behaviours: trying to bite other animals or handlers, baring teeth, teeth grinding, self-mutilation and eating foreign bodies.**

- Donkeys may die within a few days of the onset of clinical signs. However, progression can be slower (up to two weeks) in some cases.

Personal protection of any handlers, clinicians or other professionals is of utmost importance and must always be the primary consideration when examining or carrying out procedures on a donkey suspected of being infected with rabies.

> ⚠ **ALERT**
>
> Caution must always be exercised when handling or carrying out a clinical examination of an animal suspected of infection with rabies. This is especially relevant to the oral examination.

Glanders

The infectious agent is *Burkholderia* and it is found in respiratory secretions and from exudate from nodular abscesses, where they are found in the skin. Transmission is by direct contact, fomites and environmental contamination.

Clinical signs in the donkey are:

- fever

- nasal discharge

- enlarged lymph nodes

- coughing.

Note that:

- Donkeys are reported to be the most susceptible equid species.

- They will often develop the acute form of the disease and it is often fatal.

- There have been reports of outbreaks of Glanders in donkeys.

Trypanosomiasis

Trypanosoma brucei equiperdum, T. b. evansi, T. vivax, T. congolense and *T. brucei* are the most common trypanosomes infecting donkeys. Transmission is by biting insects, with the exception of *T. brucei*, which is sexually transmitted.

Trypanosomiasis is usually subclinical or chronic in donkeys.

Signs vary according to the species of trypanosomes involved, the virulence of the strain and the general health status of the animals, including level of stress, work, pregnancy status and any concurrent diseases.

Trypanosomes affecting donkeys:

Trypanosomes	Mode of transmission	Common name
Trypanosoma brucei equiperdum	Coital	Dourine
T. b. evansi	Biting flies (Tabanids)	Surra
T. vivax	Biting and tsetse flies	Nagana
T. congolense	Tsetse flies (Glossina spp)	Nagana
T. b. brucei	Tsetse flies	Nagana

Note that:

- Donkeys are generally considered more resistant to trypanosomiasis than horses and ponies.

- Studies in sub-Saharan Africa, where tsetse-transmitted trypanosomiasis is endemic, have shown high prevalence of infection and clinical cases of *T. congolense, T. b. brucei and T. vivax* (African Animal Trypanosomiasis (AAT)) in working donkeys.

- Mixed infections with two or more *Trypanosoma spp.* are common findings in donkeys, and are often fatal.

- Donkeys suffer from both patent and subclinical infections. AAT is claimed as the major health constraint of working donkeys in tsetse-belt regions of Ethiopia and Kenya.

T. b. brucei:

- Recent studies in Gambia show an increasing incidence of the neurological form.

- The disease is often fatal.

- **Clinical signs** are deteriorating cerebral function and cranial nerve abnormalities with diffuse lymphocytic-plasmacytic meningo-encephalomyelitis.

T. b. evansi (Surra):

- Surra is often reported in donkeys with a high infection prevalence and sometimes as an outbreak.

- Both acute and chronic infection with *T. b. evansi* have been reported in donkeys.

- **Clinical signs** are associated with:

  - high levels of parasitaemia

  - anaemia

  - meningoencephalitis and

  - follicular hyperplasia of lymph nodes and the spleen.

T. b. equiperdum (Dourine):

- Dourine has been reported in donkeys and typical clinical cases of Dourine are seen in the highlands of Ethiopia, where it is endemic.

- Dourine in donkeys and mules is mild to asymptomatic and may produce variable signs.

- **Clinical signs**, when evident, may include:

  - anaemia

  - oedema in the genitals (although this is often not obvious)

- skin plaques (only rarely seen)

When treating Trypanosomiasis note that:

- Over 50% of samples from donkey and mule sera show anti-complementarity. This can be reduced by dilution of the serum by half and heat inactivation at 60—63°C.

- Although trypanocidal drugs are effective in donkeys, adverse reactions are also recorded. Clinicians are therefore advised to consult local regulations and manufacturer's recommendations prior to treatment.

- Drug resistance is becoming a major problem including in donkeys and this must be taken into consideration when treating donkeys and mules in endemic areas.

Equine Piroplasmosis (EP)

The infectious agent is *Babesia* and transmission is by ticks.

EP is usually subclinical in donkeys unless other stress factors are concurrent.

Note that:

- Concurrent infection with *Theileria equi* and *Babesia caballi* is common in donkeys and is endemic in most tropical and subtropical regions.

- Although EP is usually subclincial in the donkey, **clinical signs** may be seen and include:

    - congested mucous membranes

    - lacrimation

    - depression

    - fever.

- Once infected, donkeys usually remain asymptomatic carriers with positive antibody titres throughout life.

- Stress factors, concurrent disease and reintroduction to an infected area after a period of absence may precipitate clinical infection in the donkey. Stress from poor management, inadequate veterinary care, poor nutrition and overwork, may exacerbate the impact of infection in working donkeys.

- Treatment with imidocarb diproprionate has been found to be effective.

> ⚠ **ALERT**
>
> Care must be taken to avoid the side effects of imidocarb diproprionate in the donkey especially at higher doses. Imidocarb dihydrochloride must not be used.

➡ *See chapter 17: Pharmacology and Therapeutics for more information on dosages.*

Others

Anthrax, Brucellosis, West Nile Fever, Equine encephalomyelitis and **Contagious Equine Metritis**, are all found in donkeys and treated as in horses and ponies.

OTHER INFECTIOUS DISEASES

The majority of the infectious diseases show clinical signs in donkeys similar to those seen in horses and ponies and are treated in the same way.

It is important to note that:

- Diseases that typically show signs of diarrhoea in the horse and pony may not present with diarrhoea in the donkey. Examples are Salmonella and Clostridial enterocolitis.

- Donkeys are rarely vaccinated effectively and may therefore be at an increased risk of infection; tetanus is an example.

> ⚠ **ALERT**
>
> Possible infection with diseases such as salmonella and clostridia should not be ruled out, even in the absence of diarrhoea.

Tetanus

Tetanus is a risk where donkeys have not been vaccinated effectively. This is frequently the case and prophylaxis must always be an important consideration where wounds are present.

Diagnosis and treatment is as in horses and ponies.

➡ *See Chapter 5: The Nervous System for more information.*

Strangles

Strangles is found in donkeys and is diagnosed and treated as in horses and ponies.

Commercially available serological tests for S. equi have not been validated in donkeys and therefore should be interpreted with caution.

➡ *See Chapter 4: The Respiratory System for more information.*

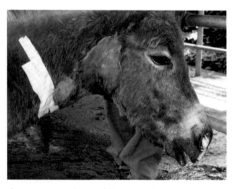

A young donkey with strangles characterised by purulent nasal discharge and enlargement of the retropharyngeal and submandibular lymph nodes.

Salmonella

Salmonella affects donkeys similarly to horses and ponies, with the exception that diarrhoea is not typically seen as a presenting sign in the donkey.

PREVENTION

Measures to control or prevent infectious diseases in donkeys are often lacking or ineffective.

All clinicians and animal health professionals play an important role in putting in place appropriate measures to minimise the risk to donkeys under their care.

The principles of best practice that apply to other equids and livestock in general can be used as guidelines.

- Although many vaccines are not licensed for donkeys and data on efficacy is often lacking effective vaccination programmes can be developed.

- Reliable accurate diagnosis is essential for treatment, effective control, and disease surveillance.

- Even when resources are limited effective biosecurity measures can be implemented.

- Isolating infected animals and quarantine with close monitoring of newly introduced equids strongly recommended.

- Good owner education and support is an essential yet often neglected part of effective disease control.

- Surveillance of notifiable diseases is carried out by the World Organisation for Animal Health (OIE).

➡ *See online at* **oie.int** *for more information on notifiable diseases.*

- Information on specific diseases and biosecurity can often be found on line on professional or government websites.

➡ *See online at* **codes.hblb.org.uk** *(Horserace Betting Levy Board) for more information on specific diseases; EVA, EIA, EHV, Dourine and Strangles.*

➡ *See online at* **aaep.org/guidelines/infectious-disease-control** *for equine focused information on disease control and biosecurity.*

Those diseases that are zoonotic must be approached with consideration of the impact on anyone coming into contact with the animal, or with the vector.

All clinicians and animal health workers are responsible for ensuring the safety and protection of all people involved with animals that might be infected with zoonotic disease.

Precautions must be considered:

- Personal protective equipment should be used where appropriate.
- Personnel should be vaccinated where appropriate and possible.
- Insect repellents and barriers should be used where appropriate.
- Prophylaxis may be necessary.

🐴 MULES AND HINNIES

The severity of the response of the mule to infectious agents varies between that seen in the donkey and that of the horse and pony.

The mule has a more acute clinical response to EIA than the donkey, but a milder response to Glanders.

For many diseases information is not available.

ℹ FURTHER INFORMATION

Factsheets, research and detailed information can be found online at: **thedonkeysanctuary.org.uk/for-professionals**

The Working Equid Veterinary Manual: **thebrooke.org/for-professionals/ working-equid-veterinary-manual**

The World Organisation for Animal Health (OIE) can be found online at **oie.int**

Horserace Betting Levy Board (HBLB), Codes of practice for certain diseases can be found online at **codes.hblb.org.uk**

The American Association of Equine Practitioners can be found online at **aaep. org/guidelines/infectious-disease-control** for information on disease control and biosecurity.

Getachew M., Alemayehu, F., Chala, C., Amare, B., Kassa, D., Burden, F., Wernery, R., and Wernery U. A cross-sectional servo-survey of some infectious diseases of working equids in central Ethiopia. *Journal of Veterinary Medicine and Animal Health*, 2014; 6: (9) 231-238.

Kumar, S., Kumar, R. and Sugimoto C. *et al* A perspective on *Theileria equi* infections in donkeys. *Japanese Journal of Veterinary Research*, 2009; 56: (4) 171-180.

Raftery, AG., Rodgers, J. and Sutton, DGM. Treatment efficacy in Equine Trypanosomosis: A prospective comparative study of three trypanocides in over 250 clinical cases in working equidae. *Journal of Equine Veterinary Science*, 2016; 39: S99.

Paweska, J.T., Volkmann, D.H., Barnard, B.J.H. and Chirnside, E.D. (1995) Sexual and in-contact transmission of asinine strain of equine arteritis virus among donkeys. *J. Clin. Micro.*,1995; 33: (12) 3296-3299.

Stringer, A.P. Infectious Diseases of Working Equids. Vet Clin Equine, 2014; 30: 695–718.

Sutton, D.G.M., Morrison, L.J., Pollock, P.J., Hahn, C., Johnston, P.E., Sharpe, S., Rogers, J. and Murray, M. Trypanosoma brucei central nervous system infection in working equidae in West Africa: an emerging disease. *Journal of Equine Veterinary Science*, 2012;32: S80-S81.

Thiemann, A. K. Respiratory disease in the donkey: A review. *Equine veterinary Education*, 2012; 24: (9) 469-478.

11. PARASITOLOGY

Perhaps one of the biggest challenges when managing parasites in donkeys is that of clinical assessment. Donkeys with significant endoparasite burdens may appear healthy and it is rare to observe the type of clinical signs (diarrhoea, weight loss, colic or poor condition) that are more common in horses and ponies.

Although donkeys can be infected by the same parasites as horses and ponies there are some notable differences in parasite dynamics and treatment regimes, the most important being the lack of anthelmintic products licensed for use in donkeys.

ECTOPARASITES

ENDOPARASITES

TREATMENT

PREVENTION

KEY POINTS

- Resistance to the majority of the available classes of equine anthelmintics has been recorded in donkeys and this should always be considered when planning treatment regimes.

- Post-treatment testing is recommended to ensure that the treatment has been fully effective.

Donkeys have different nutritional requirements and natural behaviours compared to horses and ponies. When donkeys are kept as companion animals in temperate climates they can become obese if allowed free grazing access. Grazing should therefore be restricted for much of the year, with donkeys commonly grazed at 0.1—0.2 ha/animal.

Working donkeys are often kept on small areas of land in high densities to prevent roaming or to facilitate working needs. Such stocking densities mean that larval contamination can become high on land that is not effectively managed. The donkey is a selective grazer and will not by choice graze areas soiled with dung. However, when enclosed in small areas they may graze close to or inside dunging areas, with resultant exposure to high levels of parasite challenge.

The modern anthelmintics that are available for administration to horses and ponies have been shown to be effective in donkeys, although it is important to note that resistance has been recorded to the majority of the drugs. Administer at doses determined for the horse and pony.

Many products are not licensed for use in donkeys and owners must be informed accordingly. The use of these drugs must be in accordance with local regulations for prescription of unlicensed medication. Clinicians must consult current datasheets and acknowledge the appropriate label claim for each active ingredient or brand.

⚠ **ALERT**

Most of the drugs used for parasite control are not licensed for the donkey and relevant regulations must be followed.

ECTOPARASITES

Donkeys can be affected by the same parasites as horses and ponies and are diagnosed and treated similarly.

Pediculosis, flies, pinworm, mites, stomach bots, ticks and habronemiasis are discussed in detail in the chapter on skin.

 See Chapter 8: The Skin for more information.

⚠ **ALERT**

Topical application of treatments may be affected by the dense coat of the donkey, limiting effective distribution.

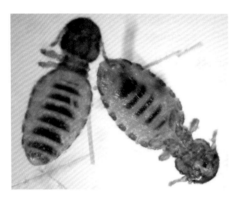

Chewing lice: the long thick coat of the donkey may hide their presence until infestation is heavy and may also hamper topical treatment.

ENDOPARASITES

Although donkeys can be infested by the same parasites as horses and ponies, it is important to note that there are some differences in parasite dynamics and in treatment regimes.

Co-grazing horses, ponies and donkeys can infect each other and this is an important consideration in the management of parasitic infestation and prevention.

Small strongyles (Cyathostomins)

As in horses and ponies, these are some of the most commonly found parasitic nematodes in donkeys globally. The donkey may not demonstrate clinical disease, particularly in populations where anthelmintics are being used.

Note that:

- Small strongyles are typically less than 1.5cm in length and excrete eggs in the faeces.

- The lifecycle of the small strongyle in donkeys is the same as in horses and ponies; the eggs develop into larvae in the soil and are then ingested and invade the wall of the large intestine.

- The period of larval encystment in the large intestinal wall plays an important role in the epidemiology and pathogenicity of infection and, because they will infect all co-grazing equids, this is an important consideration for grassland management.

- In some donkeys, encysted larvae build up in large numbers and can emerge synchronously. This may cause clinical or subclinical larval cyathostominosis.

- Donkeys do not appear to show the classical clinical signs of larval cyathostominosis and are more likely to present with weight loss, colitis and abnormally low blood proteins. It may result in colic but rarely causes diarrhoea. Mortality appears to be lower than is recorded in horses and ponies.

- Encysted larvae can persist for many months and at certain points in the year the larvae can comprise the majority of the small strongyle burden.

- Encystment is generally at a peak during the winter months in temperate climates and during the dry season in tropical climates.

- Donkeys can harbour considerable levels of infection but the parasites (encysted larvae) are not detectable by routine faecal worm egg count (FWEC) analysis.

The impact of small strongyle infections on working donkeys is unclear. Some studies indicate that they have a negative effect on body condition score and are associated with the presence of anaemia. Other studies show no correlation between FWEC and body condition score. Many donkeys appear to remain 'healthy' when high levels of small strongyles are present, as long as their health is not otherwise compromised and they are not underfed or overworked.

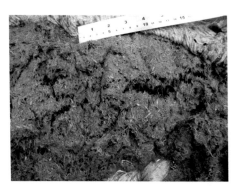 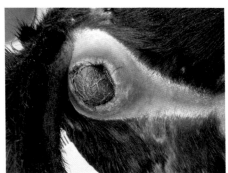

Post-mortem evidence of small strongyles.

Epidemiology and management is similar to that seen in horses and ponies, where individual animals vary in susceptibility to small strongyles. Generally, in well managed populations, the majority control their level of infection relatively well. This is demonstrated by a negative or low FWEC. Frequently, a few animals will harbour high levels of infection and will excrete moderate to high numbers of eggs into the environment. It is these individual donkeys that act as the main source of contamination with infective small strongyle larvae. It is thought, but not proven, that each donkey's relative susceptibility to small strongyle infection is maintained through life.

Small strongyle infections tend to be higher in younger donkeys, especially those grazed on permanent pastures. Mature donkeys can harbour substantial infections and therefore contribute to pasture contamination or develop disease.

The role of mature donkeys as contributors to contamination should be assessed carefully when managing foals, immunocompromised animals or mixed equine herds.

Infestation can be managed by:

- using a treatment programme that includes a once yearly larvicidal treatment – for example, moxidectin

- using seasonal FWEC to identify new infections and to assist with reducing pasture contamination. However a FWEC does not provide any information on the presence of encysted larvae, so should not be relied upon for this purpose.

The decision to treat for small strongyles (other than a once yearly treatment for encysted larvae) should be based upon a FWEC. There is no recognised threshold for treatment. In the majority of cases treatment of individuals with a FWEC equal to or greater than 300epg is reasonable.

When individual animals are routinely presenting with high FWECs, it is recommended that screening for Pars Pituitary Intermedia Dysfunction (PPID) is undertaken, because there appears to be an association with high FWECs.

When choosing drugs for treatment consider:

- All classes of drug licensed for small strongyles appear to be safe in donkeys; dose according to guidelines developed for horses and ponies.
- Moxidectin should be reserved for targeted use against encysted larvae only.
- Other drugs – for example, ivermectin and pyrantel embonate – should be considered when treatment is indicated by a FWEC.
- It should be noted that high levels of resistance to fenbendazole have been noted in the global equine population.
- Lower levels of resistance to ivermectin, moxidectin and pyrantel embonate have also been detected in donkeys parasites.
- Some classes – for example, moxidectin – are not licensed for use in donkeys and must only be prescribed according to the relevant local regulations.

> ⚠ **ALERT**
> A faecal egg count reduction test should be carried out at 14 days post treatment if there are concerns about resistance to the anthelmintic used.

Large strongyles (S equinus, vulgaris and edentatus)

Donkeys are susceptible to large strongyles with a similar lifecycle to those seen in horses.

Like small strongyles, adult worms are found in the large intestine, but the parasitic larval stages are migratory. The time from infestation to detection of eggs in faeces is in the region of 6–12 months. Otherwise, the lifecycle and epidemiology are similar to small strongyles.

> ⚠ **ALERT**
>
> Large strongyle eggs are indistinguishable from those of small strongyles so FWECs cannot be relied upon for guidance.

Large strongyle infestations remain a real threat to working donkeys and mules where administration of macrocyclic lactone anthelmintics (moxidectin and ivermectin) – is erratic or absent. *Strongylus spp.* were identified in over 90% of pooled faecal samples obtained from donkeys tested in Ethiopia and in 100% of donkeys that were examined post-mortem. Large strongyle eggs are indistinguishable from those of small strongyles, so FWECs cannot be relied upon for guidance.

When choosing the drugs for treatment, consider:

- Once-yearly administration of moxidectin for encysted small strongyles should be sufficient to control large strongyles in most populations.

- At present there is no indication of resistance to anthelmintics in the large strongyles.

- In populations where administration of anthelmintics is unknown, erratic or absent, treatment should be undertaken as a precaution.

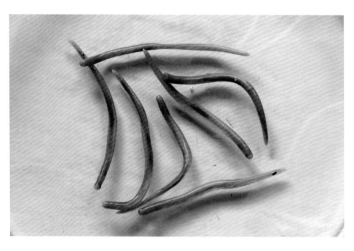

Large Strongyles.

Roundworm (*Parascaris equorum*)

Horses and ponies acquire immunity to this small intestinal nematode relatively quickly with age and exposure. Patent infections (as detected by the observation of round, thick-shelled eggs in faeces) are usually only seen in horse and pony foals.

In donkeys, mature animals harbour patent infections and otherwise healthy, mature donkeys may be important sources of pasture contamination. When compromised through overwork, ill health or poor nutrition, they may be at risk of parascaris related disease.

The life cycle of the roundworm is migratory and infection is in the form of an environmentally resistant egg containing a second stage larva. Time from infection to detection of eggs in faeces is approximately 10 weeks. The parasite is relatively common, especially in large populations where animals graze permanent pastures, and can cause clinical problems when infection intensity is high.

Roundworm eggs are extremely tolerant of environmental challenges and are known to survive for years on pastures. Assessment and treatment of new donkeys is essential. Collection and proper composting of dung is especially important on premises known to have roundworm present.

Because the migratory pattern is hepato-tracheal, respiratory signs may be observed in donkeys under high levels of challenge. Other signs include failure to thrive, whole adult worms in faeces and, in cases where infection intensity is high, direct effects on the intestine. The latter effect is rare but holds a poor prognosis.

The Donkey Sanctuary is aware of treatment failures against *P. equorum* when using ivermectin, moxidectin and pyrantel embonate in donkeys. Anthelmintic resistance should therefore be considered when designing control programmes.

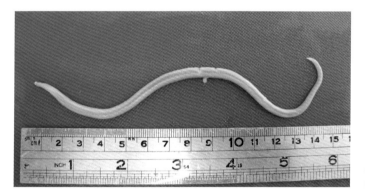

Parascaris equorum.

Pinworm *(Oxyuris equi)*
In most cases pinworm produces few or no clinical signs but persistent infection can lead to damage around the perineum and tail head.

The lifecycle and epidemiology of the pinworm in donkeys is the same as that seen in horses and ponies.

When choosing the drugs for treatment, consider:

- Anthelmintics that have demonstrated efficacy against larval and adult pinworm in horses and ponies include ivermectin, moxidectin and fenbendazole, although not all brands have a licence for this activity. pyrantel embonate has demonstrated efficacy against adult stages only.

- Pinworm appears increasingly refractory to anthelmintic treatment and The Donkey Sanctuary has reported a lack of response to treatment with both ivermectin and pyrantel embonate in donkeys. Licensed treatments include ivermectin, moxidectin and pyrantel embonate.

- It is important that good hygiene is practiced to reduce the levels of infective eggs in the environment. Thorough cleaning with a strong disinfectant after removal of all bedding will reduce the risk of infection from the environment.

- The Donkey Sanctuary uses pyrantel embonate at double the normal dose and pays particular attention to pasture, housing and animal hygiene. A second treatment with pyrantel embonate may be required as this drug is only licensed for adult pinworm.

Tapeworm (*Anoplocephala magna* and *Anoplocephala perfoliata*)

Tapeworm does not appear to be common in donkeys in temperate climates and reports of clinical disease in donkeys associated with this parasite are rare. *A. perfoliata* has been identified in 8% of working donkeys examined in Ethiopia.

This parasite has an indirect lifecycle involving an oribatid mite.

Where clinicians are aware that tapeworm is common in the local equine population, or if tapeworm eggs and/or segments are seen on faecal tests, then treatment once per year is recommended.

Faecal counts are insensitive for tapeworm and should not be relied upon for diagnosis. Similarly, ELISA-based tests have not been validated in donkeys.

When choosing the drugs for treatment consider:

- Treatment should be undertaken in late autumn or winter in temperate climates or as indicated in other climates.

- Products specifically licensed for tapeworm should be used. pyrantel embonate at an increased dose ('double dose').

- Praziquantel is not licensed for use in donkeys. It should be used where appropriate and according to relevant local regulations when pyrantel embonate is not available.

- No data is available for the use of combination de-wormers in donkeys – for example, ivermectin + praziquantel or moxidectin + praziquantel .The Donkey Sanctuary does not recommend their use.

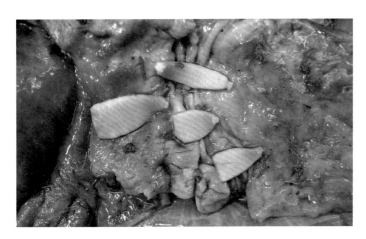

Tapeworm segments.

Threadworm *(Strongyloides westeri)*

The lifecycle and epidemiology of the threadworm in donkeys is the same as in horses and ponies.

Lungworm *(Dictyocaulus arnfieldi)*

Mature horses are not permissive hosts to the full lifecycle of this parasite, but develop clinical signs on infection. In contrast, the donkey is permissive of the entire lifecycle of the lungworm but rarely displays overt clinical signs, and also acts as a source of infection to co-grazing horses.

➜ *See Chapter 4: The Respiratory System for more information.*

Adult worms are found in the respiratory passages and eggs are coughed up and swallowed and passed out in the faeces. Note that this is different to lungworms of other host species, in which first stage larvae (L1) are usually detected in faecal samples.

Donkeys do not often exhibit clinical signs of infection, yet may excrete large numbers of eggs in their faeces. Infection in horses can cause severe coughing.

Donkeys most at risk of developing disease are those that are geriatric or immunocompromised through disease or overwork. The administration of corticosteroids or the presence of PPID appears to be correlated with higher lungworm burdens and the screening of such donkeys for lungworm infection is recommended.

Lungworm eggs hatch quickly, so diagnostic analysis should include examination for eggs by standard FWEC methods, particularly if samples are fresh and have been stored anaerobically, as well as by the Baermann technique for L1.

The control of lungworm in donkeys is particularly beneficial for co-grazing equines. It is essential to maintain a 'zero tolerance' approach to this parasite because once established on pasture it is extremely difficult to eradicate due to the ability of L3 to overwinter.

When choosing drugs for treatment, consider:

- Lungworm can be successfully treated with macrocyclic lactones.

- There is currently no indication of resistance to anthelmintics.

- A de-worming schedule that includes a once yearly larvicidal macrocyclic lactones treatment should control lungworm in closed populations.

- Newly introduced donkeys or mules should always be treated with an macrocyclic lactones and restricted from grazing for 48 hours.

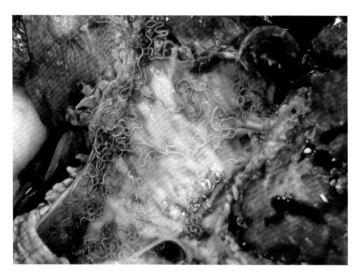

Lungworm in the respiratory passages.

Liver fluke (*Fasciola hepatica*)

Liver fluke affects mainly cattle and sheep, but can infect many mammalian species. Donkeys appear to be susceptible to liver fluke and this parasite is an increasing problem in donkeys globally. The prevalence of liver fluke infection (diagnosed by coprology) in newly admitted donkeys to The Donkey Sanctuary, UK, between 2011-2013 was 10.2%. Donkeys grazing wet, marshy paddocks are susceptible because fluke requires the water snail *Lymnaea spp.* to act as an intermediate host. Donkeys may be at particular risk if co-grazing with other infected livestock.

The adult fluke is found in the bile ducts and overt clinical signs are not usually observed in infected donkeys. Thickened bile ducts and raised levels of liver enzymes in serum may occasionally be noted in heavily infected animals.

Donkeys should have a faecal sample assessed using a sedimentation technique if fluke infestation is known to be a risk.

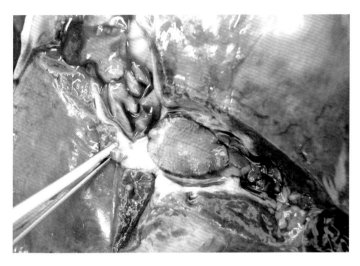

Fasciola hepatica noted at post-mortem.

Where liver fluke are known to be present in other hosts, control programmes must address the exclusion of snail habitats (by fencing or drainage), which will help break the lifecycle.

When choosing drugs for treatment, consider:

• There are no flukicidal products licensed for use in donkeys so treatment must be prescribed according to relevant local regulations.

• Triclabendazole has been used extensively by The Donkey Sanctuary at an increased dose rate of 18mg/kg bwt.

• There are numerous reports of lack of efficacy of triclabendazole and this has been observed in donkey infestations. To ensure treatment has been successful, a faecal sample should be analysed 14—28 days post treatment.

• Where triclabendazole is known to be ineffective, closantel (20mg/kg bwt) may be considered. It should be noted that this product is only effective against adult fluke so re-dosing is required 8—10 weeks later. Symptoms of closantel overdose are rare and include blindness, anorexia and ataxia. These symptoms have not been observed by The Donkey Sanctuary.

TREATMENT

⚘ DRUGS

Anthelmintics available for use in treating helminth infections in donkeys in the UK			
Anthelmintic class	Active ingredient	Indication	Dose rate
Macrocyclic lactones	Ivermectin	GI nematodes, *Dictyocaulus arnfieldi*	0.2mg/kg bwt per os
	Moxidectin*	As above + encysted cyathostomin larvae	0.4mg/kg bwt per os
Benzimidazoles	Fenbendazole†	GI nematodes, *D. arnfieldi*	7.5mg/kg bwt per os or 7.5mg/kg bwt per os for 5 days for cyathostomin encysted larvae
	Triclabendazole*	*Immature and mature Fasciola hepatica*	18mg/kg bwt
Tetrahydropyrimidines	Pyrantel embonate	Gastrointestinal nematodes	19mg/kg bwt
		Anoplocephala perfoliatia	38mg/kg bwt
Pyrozinoisoquinolines	Praziquantel*	*A. perfoliatia* and other tapeworms	2.5mg/kg bwt
Salicylanilides	Closantel*	Mature *F. hepatica*	20mg/kg bwt

* Not licensed for use in donkeys. Prescribe according to relevant local regulations.
† High levels of resistance to this anthelmintic reported in cyathostomins, worldwide.

Early studies indicate that the reappearance period for strongyle eggs are shorter in donkeys than in horses and ponies.

The first report of moxidectin resistance in equine small strongyles was recorded in donkeys.

PREVENTION

It is imperative that preventative programmes balance parasite control with the requirement to preserve anthelmintic effectiveness.

Environmental management

Anthelmintics reduce pasture contamination and treat clinical disease but only impact on parasites within the animal. The vast majority of parasites reside in the environment. This includes buildings or fences in some cases. Control of the environmental population is essential.

Simple control measures include:

- Dung removal at least twice per week has been shown to significantly decrease the number of parasite larvae present and the requirement to treat with anthelmintics. This is especially important when equids are intensively grazed.

- Manure should be properly composted before being spread on to grazing land. Manure should be composted for a minimum of six weeks with regular turning and maintenance. A minimum temperature of 50—70°C is recommended to kill helminth eggs.

- New equines should be quarantined and treated. Treatment for lungworm with an macrocyclic lactones is recommended for any new donkey or mule entering a property before it is allowed to graze.

- Co-grazing with ruminants is useful as a 'biological hoover'. Care should be taken grazing donkeys alongside other species as they can exhibit aggressive behaviour towards unknown animals; unless they are carefully introduced, grazing separately is recommended.

- Disinfection of stables, fencing and fomites is advisable where *Parascaris* or *Oxyuris* are present.

- Where fluke is an issue, drainage of grazing land and treatment and monitoring of other livestock is strongly recommended.

🐴 MULES AND HINNIES

Mules have an intermediate susceptibility to *Dictyocaulus arnfieldi*. Mules may rarely support a patent infection and are more likely than donkeys to exhibit clinical signs associated with infestation. Preventative testing and treatment should be followed as for donkeys.

ℹ️ FURTHER INFORMATION

Factsheets, research and detailed information can be found online at:
thedonkeysanctuary.org.uk/for-professionals

Burden, F.A and Getachew, M. (2016). Donkeys – a unique and challenging endoparasite host. *Journal of Equine Veterinary Science.* 39:S102–S103.

Burden, F.A. and Trawford, A.F. Donkeys' parasites in the UK: Infection levels, treatment intervals and anthelmintic use. *22nd International Conference of the Worldwide Association for the Advancement of Veterinary Parasitology.* (9 August – 13 August 2009). Calgary, Canada.

Getachew A. M., Innocent, G.T., Trawford, A.T., Feseha, G., Reid, S.J.W. and Love, S. (2008). Equine parascarosis under the tropical weather conditions of Ethiopia: a coprological and postmortem study. *Veterinary Record.* 162:6. 177-180

Getachew, M. (2006) *Endoparasites of working donkeys in Ethiopia: epidemiological study and mathematical modelling.* PhD thesis, University of Glasgow.

Matthews, J.B. and Burden, F.A. (2013) Common helminth infections of donkeys and their control in temperate regions. *Equine Veterinary Education,* 25:461-467. doi:10.1111/eve12018

Matthews, J.B. (2008) An update on cyathostomins: anthelmintic resistance and worm control. *Equine Veterinary Education.* 20, 552-560. doi:10.2746/095777308X363912

Trawford, A.F., Burden, F. and Hodgkinson, J.E. (2005) Suspected moxidectin resistance in cyathostomes in two donkey herds at the Donkey Sanctuary, UK. *20th International Conference of the World Association for the Advancement of Veterinary Parasitology,* New Zealand. pp 196.

12. APPROACH TO THE DULL DONKEY

Many people wrongly assume that the donkey's normal behaviours are less expressive than those seen in horses and ponies and do not appreciate that a healthy donkey should not appear dull. The donkey will still suffer from pain but the survival strategy of this prey species is to mask the obvious signs of pain. Subtle changes in a donkey's behaviour may indicate severe pain and serious disease. Dull companion or pet donkeys are most likely to be suffering from impaction colic, pain and/or hyperlipaemia. Dull or apathetic working donkeys may be suffering from multiple problems, including exhaustion.

Therefore, any donkey exhibiting subtle changes in normal behaviour and appetite, or with a dull demeanour, should be examined thoroughly and urgently to detect the underlying cause(s).

The dull donkey should be included in the vet's list of equine emergencies.

Supportive treatment can be provided until a diagnosis can be made.

NORMAL BEHAVIOUR

PAIN RELATED BEHAVIOURS

CLINICAL EXAMINATION

TREATMENT

PAIN MANAGEMENT

PREVENTION

KEY POINTS

- Normal, healthy pain free donkeys should exhibit a wide range of behaviours and interactions with people and other animals.

- A donkey showing signs of social isolation, withdrawal and apathy may be very sick.

- Subtle signs of pain/changes in behaviour should prompt a veterinary examination.

- As pain behaviours may be non-specific a detailed clinical examination including rectal examination and blood sampling should be carried out.

- Supportive treatment for a dull donkey should include analgesia at appropriate doses and nutritional management to avoid hyperlipaemia.

PREVENTION

- Avoid sudden changes in feed or management where possible.

- Adopt effective programmes of preventative care to lower the risk of illness.

- Avoid seperation from companion/s.

NORMAL BEHAVIOUR

Donkeys often live to advanced ages or in many countries are worked/overworked to near exhaustion. For these reasons the common perception is that all donkeys tend to look dull or quiet. There can be a lack of appreciation of the normal full range of behaviours that healthy, pain free donkeys engage in.

Familiarity with the normal behaviour of a donkey allows identification of subtle changes in behaviour and demeanour and earlier awareness of problems.

➔ *See Chapter 1: Behaviour for more information.*

Young donkeys in particular, should be friendly, inquisitive and playful. Mature donkeys should still engage in behaviours such as mutual grooming, exploring new items, and being part of a group.

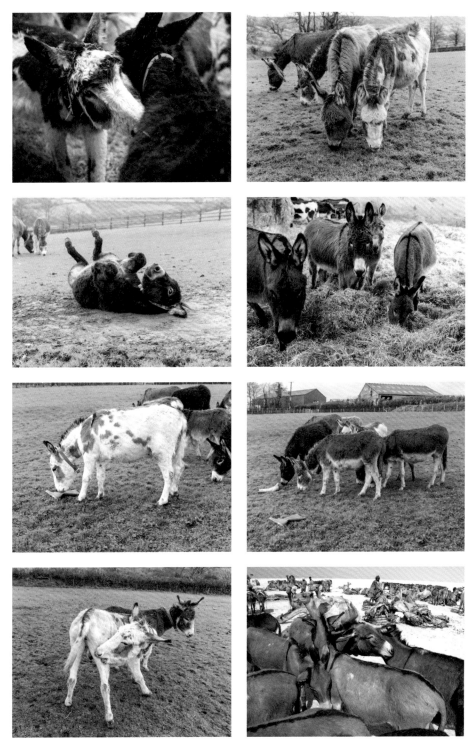

Healthy young donkeys and adult donkeys exhibiting normal behaviour.
Absence of these behaviours is an indication of the dull donkey.

Healthy donkeys will have a good appetite for forage, browsing and treats, and will chew excessively at wooden fences or logs if deprived of fibre.

In response to thermal stress a healthy donkey will shiver and try to find shelter if cold, and seek shade if too hot.

As befits a herbivore and prey animal, a donkey should spend most of its day (12-20 hours) foraging over wide distances. It may sleep lying down, in short bouts (of approximately 15 minutes for a total of 2-6 hours), and relax standing up for approximately 2-6 hours while another member of its group is on guard.

Studies show that healthy donkeys do exhibit a wide range of behaviours relating to moving, resting, interacting with each other and the environment, and that by being familiar with these the observer can assess and understand when the donkey is in pain or unwell (Regan *et al*, 2014).

> ⚠ **ALERT**
>
> Early identification of subtle changes in behaviour and demeanour is essential for earlier awareness of problems.

PAIN RELATED BEHAVIOURS

By understanding these normal behaviours, it follows that an absence of these is a clue that the donkey may be in some form of pain or distress. If the owners of a donkey are only used to the behaviours exhibited by the small companion animals then there is potential for delayed recognition of serious problems. For example the prolonged recumbency of a donkey with colic or laminitis is not comparable to the resting behaviour of a dog, and the self-isolation of a sick donkey is not comparable to the normal solitary state preferred by many cats.

Detailed observational studies of working donkeys have shown that using pain relief improved general alertness and inquisitive behaviours and resulted in a higher head position and less restlessness. Donkeys were seen to rest more and show fewer weight shifting behaviours (Regan *et al*, 2014).

In contrast, when donkeys are overworked and exhausted with severe physical problems they may "shut down", showing apathy and a very limited range of behaviours. Animals in such a state have severely compromised welfare, although it may not be easily apparent which system is primarily involved.

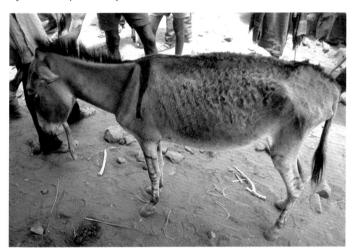

Exhausted "switched off" behaviour of working donkey.

Further studies asked clinicians familiar with donkeys to rate pain prior to euthanasia, and this was correlated with the presence of previously ascribed painful lesions at post-mortem examination (Olmos & Burden, 2012). This study found that up to 20% of donkeys were incorrectly identified as not being in pain, and that several subtle behaviours were not being recognised and acted upon by the clinicians.

Some important findings were that donkeys in pain:

* spent more time than controls with lowered head carriage

- had ears that were more static and unresponsive to changes in the environment

- spent up to 30% more time recumbent

- spent up to 40% less time eating.

Pain related behaviours in the donkey can be divided into general and system specific behaviours. The general behaviours of a dull donkey are to show a reduced normal behaviour repertoire and those found to be relating to pain include symptoms such as:

- general depression

- reduced interactions and self-isolation and a lack of social grooming

- lowered ears, ears that fail to move independently to stimuli, ears often being held horizontally or facing rearward

- lowered head and neck; they may be held below withers height

- ineffective (or sham) eating or drinking

- inappetence

- anxiety

- abnormal aggression

- reluctance to move with less general movement.

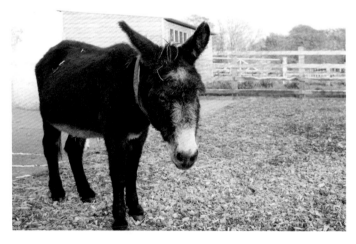

Typical head down, ears back posture of donkey in pain.

System specific pain behaviours tend to be less obvious than in horses and ponies.

- While lameness is evident with limb or hoof pain, it is also common for donkeys to lie down more and show reluctance to move.

- With abdominal pain it is more common for donkeys to show

inappetence and recumbency rather than rolling and kicking at the abdomen.

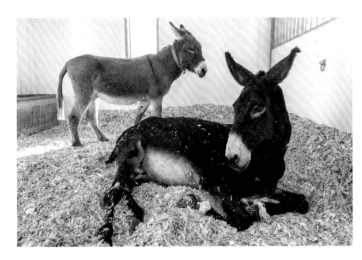

Recumbent donkey – is it lame, suffering colic, or just resting?

Research is being directed at the ability to detect pain in donkeys using a modified Horse Grimace Scale. Early results appear promising.

CLINICAL EXAMINATION

Analgesia and supportive therapy, including fluids and nutrition, are the most important first-line treatments for a dull donkey. A detailed investigation for a final diagnosis of the problem can follow.

A study on the causes of dullness in a herd of donkeys found that colic and hyperlipaemia accounted for over a third of cases presented. Lameness, liver disease and respiratory disorders were the next most prevalent causes identified. There was a long list of diseases that accounted for non-specific dullness in the donkeys, including all organ systems (Theimann, 2013).

Due to the wide range of conditions that may present with subtle signs when a donkey is ill, a full detailed clinical examination is needed for diagnosis. This should include a rectal examination, a full mouth examination with a oral speculum, and a blood sample to check for hyperlipaemia.

➜ *See Appendix 1 for a summary of the Clinical Examination.*

If it is not clear which system is involved in dullness, then a full blood screen should be run, particularly to assess hepatic and renal function.

➜ *See Appendix 4 for the normal haematology and biochemistry reference ranges.*

The difficulties with carrying out a rectal examination in a small patient can be overcome by the use of good restraint and sedation if necessary. Good lubrication will aid the procedure and spasmolytic medication can be used at the standard equine dose where this is appropriate. In cases where this is really not possible an ultrasound examination of the abdomen may be needed.

➜ *See Chapter 3: The Gastrointestinal System for more information on the examination and treatment of a donkey with colic.*

Key points in the examination of a dull donkey include:

* Observe behaviours including attitude to eating before examining.
* Check history, including any possible recent (within previous 2 weeks) stressors such as changes in diet, management or loss of companions.
* Check vaccination status, deworming history and dental care records; many donkeys have poor, or absent, preventative health programmes.
* Keep closely bonded pairs of donkeys together for examination and treatment where possible.
* Be aware of normal donkey specific physiological parameters.
* A full clinical examination should include rectal and oral examination.

- Respiratory examination may need to include a re-breathing bag due to the non-athletic nature of the donkey.

- A lameness examination, including mobility assessment, may be difficult, donkeys may follow companions more easily than being led.

Donkeys can live to a marked old age, and it can be challenging to ascribe new pain related behaviours to a geriatric donkey that has age related conditions. For example, many older donkeys are maintained on medication to allow long term comfort in cases of osteoarthritis or low grade lameness. These animals may be even more challenging to diagnose and treat in a timely fashion.

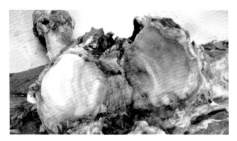

Severe osteoarthritis of shoulder in a 12 year old donkey managed on NSAIDs.

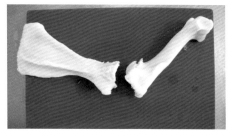

The severity of the disease suggests that the donkey would have been in severe discomfort despite the medication.

The use of objective assessments for the quality of life to monitor the aged donkey is a valuable tool in determining when to change medication and management, or to consider euthanasia.

➔ *See Chapter 14: The Geriatric Donkey for more information and Appendices 5 and 6 for quality of life monitoring templates.*

TREATMENT

In many cases the primary cause of the dullness or pain may not be readily apparent. The first aim should be to stabilise and support the patient, provide adequate analgesia, and plan to re-examine and perform further tests at an appropriate interval.

Donkeys with depressed appetite, ineffective ('sham') eating or anorexia, can be assumed to be hyperlipaemic or on the way to becoming so. Fluid and nutritional support is required either by naso-gastric intubation or intravenously (if ileus is present).

It is good practice to provide this prior to blood results becoming available to avoid delays in treatment.

➔ *See Chapter 7: Hyperlipaemia and the Endocrine System for more information.*

These patients will also need gastric protectants as they are at high risk of developing gastric ulceration.

PAIN MANAGEMENT

Analgesia at a dosage and frequency that is appropriate for the donkey should be given. The response to treatment must be evaluated regularly.

- Many of the commonly used NSAIDs will need to be given at a higher dosing rate as the donkey has a different drug metabolism to that in horses and ponies.

- Adjunct analgesia may be required but there is little or no donkey specific data.

- Use opioids, ketamine, lidocaine, paracetamol at quoted equine dose rates, and monitor quality of analgesia.

- Fentanyl patches may need changing more frequently in the donkey.

- Local anaesthetic blocks should be used where possible - for example, for dental extractions, castration or lameness.

➡ *See Chapter 17: Pharmacology and Therapeutics and Chapter 16: Sedation, Anaesthetics and Analgesia for more information.*

Many donkeys respond well to good nursing care and this can be difficult to provide in a standard equine hospital. For example stable doors are too high for donkeys to see over but a solution may be to use gates or hurdles in place of the door.

Improving the mental well-being of the sick donkey is important for recovery:

- Keep the companion nearby.

- Maintain a calm environment.

- Allow access to grazing if possible.

PREVENTION

In the majority of cases the donkey only demonstrates subtle indications of pain or changes in behaviour and may only show obvious signs in the advanced stages of a condition or when suffering severe pain. Therefore, the dull donkey is often an emergency.

If donkey owners learn to regularly assess their donkey's normal behaviour patterns, they can be quick to respond to any subtle changes indicating dullness.

The regular use of good up-to-date programmes of preventative health care will help reduce the incidence of many problems. Most important are:

- parasite control
- dental examinations and care
- foot care
- weight control
- vaccination.

It cannot always be achieved but care should be taken to reduce stressful situations, and this includes changes to feeding and management. Where possible, changes should be made slowly and the health of the donkey monitored throughout.

🐴 MULES AND HINNIES

There is very limited information and evidence available for the mule and therefore nothing to add that is specific to the mule.

ℹ️ FURTHER INFORMATION

Factsheets, research and detailed information can be found online at: **thedonkeysanctuary.org.uk/for-professionals**

Regan, F.H., Hockenhull, J., Pritchard, J.C., Waterman- Pearson, A.E. and Whay, H.R. (2014) Behavioural repertoire of working donkeys and consistency of behaviour over time, as a preliminary step towards identifying pain- related behaviours. *PLoSOne*, Jul 30, 9 (7): e101877.

Regan, F.H., Hockenhull. J., Pritchard, J.C., Waterman-Pearson A.E., and Whay H.R., (2016) Identifying behavioural differences in working donkeys in response to analgesic administration *Equine Vet Journal* 48 (1) 33-38.

Ashley, F.H., Waterman-Pearson, A.E. and Whay, H.R. (2005) Behavioural assessment of pain in horses and donkeys: application to clinical practice and future studies. *Equine Veterinary Journal* 37, 565-575.

Olmos, G., Burden, F.A. (2012). A novel approach to pain recognition in donkeys. Presented at 14th World Congress on Pain, Satellite Symposia: Pain and Pain Management in Non-Human Species. (27 August - 31 August 2012). Milan, Italy.

Thiemann, A.K. (2013).Clinical approach to the dull donkey. *In Practice* 35, 470-476.

13. THE CARE OF THE FOAL

Neonate survival is described as a major problem among working donkeys globally.

Risk factors for the survival of the neonatal donkey foal are similar to those for horses and ponies but consideration of the donkey specific differences could improve the survival rate and future health of the donkey.

The lack of preventative care for many female donkeys during pregnancy is an important factor. Programmes for vaccination and parasite control are essential during the pregnancy and an appropriate diet for the pregnant animal is necessary.

ROUTINE CARE OF THE NEWBORN FOAL

COMMON CONDITIONS OF THE NEWBORN FOAL

THE REJECTED AND ORPHAN FOAL

WEANING

KEY POINTS

- Pregnant and lactating donkeys are at a higher risk of hyperlipaemia. Feed must be adjusted accordingly.

- Transportation of female donkeys in the last trimester may cause unnecessary stress and increase the risk of hyperlipaemia.

- Hyperlipaemia will adversely affect milk production and colostrum quality.

- Due to the small size of the donkey foal, an accurate estimation of weight is essential, especially when calculating doses for medication.

PREVENTION

- Pregnant donkeys require a programme of vaccination, parasite control and an appropriate diet.

- Reference should be made to the donkey specific parameters when dealing with both the dam and the foal.

ROUTINE CARE OF THE NEWBORN FOAL

A foaling kit must be available during parturition.

A complete equine foaling / foal care kit is necessary, including commercial colostrum and minimum temperature thermometer capable of monitoring the significantly low temperatures that donkey foals may exhibit, with the following additional items specifically for donkeys:

- a male urinary catheter for stomach tubing

- a small iv catheter – for example, size 20—22g

- a large dog size thermal rug or blanket.

Horse milk replacer can be used for donkeys.

> ⚠ **ALERT**
>
> **Accurate weight estimation is essential for medication.**

Donkey foals tend to be lighter than the average horse or pony foal, although weight varies between individuals and breeds, ranging from 5—40kg. It is essential to estimate weight accurately when planning medication.

Note the different physiological parameters for the newborn foal.

> **ⓘ INFORMATION**
>
> **Newborn donkey physiological parameters**
>
> - **Temperature:** 37.5—38.5°C,
>   99.5—101.3°F
>
> - **Pulse:** 80—120 beats/minute in the first few hours
>
> - **Respiration:** 60—80 breaths/minute in first hour;
>   30—40 breaths/minute after 12 hours

Despite their thick coat, donkey foals are not very cold tolerant, becoming chilled rapidly if they remain wet. Therefore it is advisable to plan breeding accordingly, to avoid extreme conditions of cold, rain and heat where possible. Access to effective shelter is important.

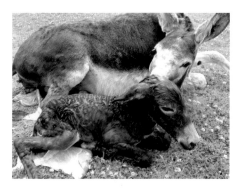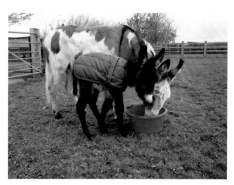

The foal's capacity for thermoregulation is limited and they may be prone to hypothermia.

Physiological differences

Donkeys have specific physiological differences to horses and ponies and these affect drug distribution and metabolism. These also apply to the donkey neonate.

In the absence of specific pharmaceutical information, drugs and dosages considered appropriate for horse and pony foals and lactating mares can be applied to donkeys.

COMMON CONDITIONS OF THE NEWBORN FOAL

The common conditions seen in newborn donkey foals are similar to those seen in horse and pony foals, but the donkey specific differences need to be considered.

Prematurity

The donkey has a variable gestation period with a reported average length of 365—376 days with a range of 11 - 14.5 months. Therefore it can be difficult to classify a donkey foal as either:

- **premature** – ie born early according to stage of gestation
- **dysmature** – ie a foal whose maturity is not appropriate for its gestational age.

Clinical signs of prematurity are similar to those found in horses and ponies. These donkeys are also prone to failure of passive immunity transfer and other disorders.

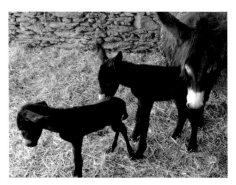
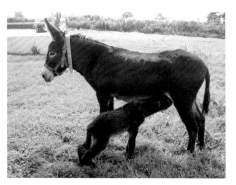

The long foal ears can be used as a good health indicator. Low muscular tone with lateral or backward position is a sign of weakness, pain or depression. The foal here was born premature at 335 days.

Premature or dismature foal, born with hyperflexion of the joints.

Meconium retention

The clinical signs and treatment of meconium retention in donkeys are similar to those in horses and ponies. Additional therapy including fluids, analgesics and laxatives by nasogastric tube can also be used in the donkey. Care must be taken when using a nasogastric tube due to the smaller size. A male urinary catheter can be used as a nasogastric tube.

Failure of passive immune transfer (FPIT)

FPIT can be found in donkey foals as a result of poor colostrum quality and/ or quantity, or inability of the newborn donkey foal to suckle. Pregnant donkeys in the last trimester and lactating donkeys have a high risk of developing hyperlipemia. This will have an adverse effect on colostrum quality and milk production. This will increase the risk of FPIT.

> ⚠ **ALERT**
>
> Donkeys have a high risk of developing hyperlipaemia in the last tremester of pregnancy. This may affect the quality of colostrum and increase the risk of FPIT.

Early treatment of FPIT is usually effective if the suckle reflex is present and good-quality colostrum is available.

If good quality colostrum is available and the foal has a good suckle reflex, bottle feeding can be used, either for supplementary feeding or for all the feed if the dam rejects the foal.

If the foal does not have a suckle reflex or does not take enough colostrum, nasogastric intubation should be used to supplement the colostrum. It is preferable to collect this from the dam but frozen colostrum can be used. If neither is available, commercial horse colostrum can be used.

Risk factors are similar to those in the horse and pony, with an incidence of up to 40% reported. Ig G concentrations considered normal in horse and pony foals are also used for the donkey foal.

Points to watch for are:

- Average sized foals should consume 1—2 litres of colostrum, depending on their size, within the first 12 hours of life.

- The first feed should be within 2—4 hours of birth.

- The recommended amount is approximately 250mls every hour for the first six hours, making a total of 1.5 litres.

- Absorption rapidly falls to less than 25% efficiency by three hours of age. Foals should be encouraged to nurse as soon as possible, whilst considering the need to maintain the bond between the dam and foal.

Supplementary colostrum should be obtained within two days of giving birth. Alternatively, frozen colostrum can be used.

Colostrum quality can be assessed with a refractometer (a specific gravity greater than 1.080 and/or a Brix score greater than or equal to 20%).

If colostrum is not available, commercial horse colostrum can be used.

Plasma transfusion is recommended if no adequate passive transfer is verified after the 24 hours post-partum, and after 12 hours in selected cases. Although expensive, hyperimmune plasma transfusion should be considered in the treatment of FPIT in donkey foals – for example, using hyperimmune plasma from Veterinary Immunogenics. Estimate the weight of the foal accurately to ensure appropriate volumes are given.

➡ *See online at **veterinaryimmunogenics.com** for website.*

In the experience of The Donkey Sanctuary, IgG levels directly compare to those found in horses and the same approach should be taken when IgG is less than 800 mg/dl. Supplementation with plasma has been very successful after only one administration, although more than one administration has been reported to be needed (repeated transfusion has been reported to be safe). Ig G levels can be checked 8—12 hours after birth, although 16—20 hours after birth has been effective.

Parameters for levels of IgG in the donkey foal	
Foal IgG concentrations (mg/dl)	Interpretation
≥ 800	Optimal passive transfer
400—800	Adequate passive transfer
200—400	Partial failure of passive transfer
< 200	Complete failure of passive transfer

Catheter placement and administration of plasma is facilitated by sedating the foal. Good levels of sedation in the donkey foal have been achieved with diazepam I/V at 0.1—0.25mg/kg. Keeping the dam occupied with a small feed may be helpful, as she might be very protective of the foal.

To carry out nasogastric intubation in a donkey foal:

- A male urinary catheter 20F (Portex) might be preferable to a horse foal nasogastric tube.

- Ensure the end is capped to avoid aerophagia.

- Nasogastric tubing in donkey foals is also a risk factor for gastric ulceration and the use of omeprazole may be indicated.

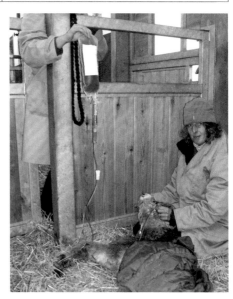

Plasma transfusion in the foal is often successful.

Neonatal septicaemia and diarrhoea

Presentation, clinical signs and treatment are the same as in the horse and pony, with problems of dysmaturity, hypothermia and FPIT potentially occuring in the same individual. Nutritional support, fluid therapy and gastric ulcer preventative treatment follow standard equine practice.

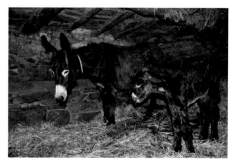

A foal with FPIT that was rejected by the mother.

Gastric ulcers

The prevalence of gastric ulcers in foals has been reported to be between 25—57%. Risk factors and clinical signs are comparable to those in horses.

Prevention and treatment with omeprazole and/or sucralfate at the standard equine dosage is appropriate. The use of omeprazole is not licensed for foals less than four weeks old or weighing less than 70kg. However, its effective use has been extensively reported.

Congenital anomalies

Anomalies of the head and jaw have been observed in donkey foals. These may affect suckling and have consequences for dystocia.

White muscle disease

Adult donkeys can be affected but foals are more susceptible to nutritional muscular dystrophy from selenium and vitamin E deficiency. Clinical signs are the same as those found in horses and ponies. Treatment and prevention can be achieved using standard equine doses of selenium in the donkey foals and by supplementation of selenium in the female donkeys.

THE REJECTED AND ORPHAN FOAL

A female donkey may show antagonistic behaviour towards her foal after birth. Common predisposing factors are:

- pain – for example, mastitis.

- behavioural problems related to fear, which may be attributed to the human presence and due to inappropriate behaviour or interference.

- previous rejection of a foal.

Providing owners are aware of this, prevention is sometimes possible.

Rejected foals are in danger of being severely injured.

Time is essential because the foal must have an early supply of colostrum followed by a regular milk supply. A foal that doesn't suckle in the early stages of life will lose the instinct to do so.

Overcoming rejection of a foal is not easy and may be impossible. The chances of success are poor if the foal is not accepted within the initial 10—12 hours after birth.

Some useful strategies are:

- The dam and foal should be in a calm environment and separated by a partition that allows them to see and smell each other.

- The dam and foal should be put together when the foal is hungry and the dam has a full udder.

- Allow the dam and foal to meet at frequent intervals, but take care to avoid negative behaviours during the meetings.

- Positive reinforcement of the dam using treats may result in a calming effect, but in some cases may cause more anxiety.

- A strong smell (for example Vicks VapoRub) placed over the dam's nostrils and on the foal, especially on head, neck and hindquarters, may help.

- Chemical tranquilisation or hobbles may be used, but the need should diminish at each subsequent meeting.

Foster mothers are the best solution for orphan foals but are rarely available. Foster mothers may include donkeys:

- whose foal died or has been weaned

- who are already feeding a foal

- in whom lactation is induced.

A donkey that has just lost her foal is the best candidate for orphan foal fostering, but fostering can also be successful using donkeys who have been weaned.

Success is increased where:

- the donkey has suckled her dead foal, and the period between foal death and orphan foal introduction is short; after 2—3 days the donkey's milk may dry up

- the donkey is moved to an alternative stable that she does not associate with her dead foal

- the amnion, meconium or hide from the dead foal is smeared over the orphan before the orphan is presented to the female donkey; in herd situations amnions and/or meconium can be usefully frozen in advance for this purpose.

A female donkey may not accept a second foal when she is already feeding. If she does it is important to consider nutritional supplementation of both the female donkey and the foal(s). Foals can be given access to a milk replacer – for example, in a bucket.

Patience and continued attempts may be needed before adoption will occur. It is possible to make an extremely hostile donkey a good mother.

Protocol for hand rearing

The successful hand rearing of donkey foals follows the same principles as for horses and ponies. Ensure a donkey companion is present at all times to avoid behavioural problems later in life.

Fresh donkey milk is preferable but, if unavailable, horse or goat milk or horse milk replacer should be used.

With regard to the frequency and volume of milk, consideration should be given to the following:

- Milk should be warmed to 38°C for initial feeds, gradually reducing to air temperature over the first week.

- Diet changes should always be made slowly over 24 to 48 hours.

- A 10kg foal requires 30kcal/kg (125kJ/kg) per day, while a sick or premature foal requires 36kcal/kg (150kJ/kg) per day.

- The recommended volume of milk for a healthy foal is 100ml/kg bw per day (10% of its body weight).

- During the first week it is preferable to feed every 1—2 hours because in natural conditions the foal would nurse from their mother an average of five times per hour, in periods of 1—2 minutes at a time. A sick foal may be unable to tolerate more than half the normal quantity per feeding, so more frequent feeding is required.

- Foals usually do not overeat but caution is recommended. Milk should be given in small quantities and often, because an excessive quantity of milk in one meal may swamp the digestive enzyme system and acidity of the stomach, leading to proliferation of pathogenic enteric microorganisms.

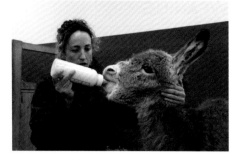

Milk should be given in small quantities and often.

- Only use recently prepared fresh milk, or powdered, to avoid bacteria development. Hands and utensils should be kept clean.

A suggested hand rearing protocol:

	Frequency	**Feed and quantity**
Day 1 & 2	Feed every 2 hours A total of 10—12 feeds a day	10—15% of body weight per feed
Day 3—7	Feed every 2—3 hours A total of 8 feeds a day	25% of body weight per feed Milk-based pellets can start being offered
Week 2	Feed every 4 hours A total of 6 feeds a day	30% of body weight per feed Allow access to fresh water and salt. Bucket feeding may be possible with some training
Week 3	Feed 6 times a day	The foal should have access to a limited quantity of good-quality hay/haylage and access to grazing. The Donkey Sanctuary recommends a supplementation with creep feed of 18% protein, with slow increases up to 100g/100kg
Week 4	Feed 5 times a day	Start omitting the night time feeding gradually
Week 8—12	Feed 4 times a day at 8 weeks Feed 3 times a day at 12 weeks	
5 months		Foals can be fully weaned at this age, but not before

Be aware that nutritional diarrhoea and lactose intolerance may occur in donkeys. Management and treatment is the same as for horses and ponies.

WEANING

At The Donkey Sanctuary we recommend weaning around a year old, when castration of male foals is also recommended . Castration is normally carried out at 10—18 months of age but might need to be considered earlier in some cases if sexual behaviour is exhibited, testicles are fully descended, or the male is living with female donkeys. Overproduction of donkey foals has been seen in many European countries and is a serious welfare problem.

Different weaning options have been reported for horses and ponies and these can be employed for donkeys. Each method has its respective merits and drawbacks. Whichever option is followed, it is important to monitor closely to avoid excessive stress and prevent the risk of hyperlipaemia. Although the feeding requirements of the female donkey will be reduced, offering extra feeds for a period of time might be of benefit.

🐴 MULES AND HINNIES

Mule foals must be monitored for neonatal isoerythrolysis because 10% of mule foals are at risk. Nearly all cases are mule foals from mares that have produced previous mule foals. Multi-parturient mares can be tested for the antidonkey red cell antibodies (donkey factor) 2—3 weeks before foaling. These foals will need to have an alternative source of colostrum and not be allowed to nurse the dam for 24—36 hours; the milk should be stripped and disposed of to prevent nursing. Once the colostrum is gone, the mare can raise the foal safely.

ⓘ FURTHER INFORMATION

Factsheets, research and detailed information can be found online at
thedonkeysanctuary.org.uk/for-professionals

Aronoff N. 2010. The Donkey Neonate. In: Veterinary Care of donkeys, Matthews N.S. and Taylor T.S. (Eds).International Veterinary information Service, Ithaca NY(www.ivis.org).Last updated 29-Mar 2010.

Hagstrom D.J (2004) Donkeys are different: an overview of reproductive variations from horses. University of Illinois/U.S. Department of Agriculture/ local extension councils cooperating.

Matthews N., Taylor T., Blanchard T (2003). An Overview of Reproduction in Donkeys. International animal health news. A publication of Christian Veterinary Mission. Vol 18 August 2003.

14. THE GERIATRIC DONKEY

Old age is inevitable but should not be uncomfortable.

The definition used for a 'geriatric' donkey is one that is over 20 years old. Many donkeys living as companions, rather than feral or working individuals, will live far beyond this age and have a long, fulfilling life. They deserve special care.

This most stoic of species represents a challenge for the clinician even though many problems faced by the geriatric donkey are similar to those seen in horses and ponies. The mixture of lifestyle, lack of monetary value and stoicism, often compounded by the lack of vigilant management experienced by many donkeys, frequently result in the occurrence of significant unrecognised disease. The geriatric donkey tends to 'suffer in silence'. Poor body condition may be veiled beneath the thick coat and common pathologies such as foot, dental, respiratory and liver disease and insulin dysregulation often go unnoticed or undiagnosed in the non-athletic individual.

An important consideration when deciding on treatment or control will be the quality of life of the donkey, both at the time of presentation and going forward. Unrecognised disease, or even controlled recognised conditions, may lead to pain and distress. Unremitting pain, anxiety or chronic discomfort will inevitably impair the donkey's quality of life. Euthanasia should be seen as a positive tool in the veterinarian's 'welfare kit' and may be the best outcome for a geriatric donkey in chronic discomfort or one that an owner is no longer able to keep.

This chapter concentrates on conditions commonly seen as a result of longevity and lifestyle. Other conditions which cannot be ruled out of the differential diagnosis can be found in other chapters.

CLINICAL EXAMINATION

COMMON CONDITIONS

GERIATRIC MANAGEMENT

ASSESSMENT OF QUALITY OF LIFE

KEY POINTS

- Donkeys are very stoic in nature. Pain behaviour is more subtle than in the horse and pony.

- Quality of Life is an important consideration.

- **The 'dull donkey' should be considered a veterinary emergency.**

- Many non-working donkeys live to old age and are likely to suffer from a range of chronic diseases.

PREVENTION

- Euthanasia should be viewed as a positive welfare outcome where quality of life is impaired despite veterinary intervention.

- Always consider the companion donkey when euthanasia is planned.

Companion donkeys are frequently managed by 'benign neglect' - although cared for in the eyes of the owners, they simply live out their lives in paddocks. Because they are not usually in work, problems that may be recognised in the ridden horse or pony may go unobserved in the donkey. For example, weight change, stiffness, or foot and dental disease may all be obvious in horses and ponies at the time of grooming, tacking up and riding.

Old age issues are frequently neglected in working donkeys around the world, with infirm animals struggling to carry loads. Sensitivity towards local cultural norms and beliefs as well as an awareness of financial, professional and practical constraints are needed when addressing these problems.

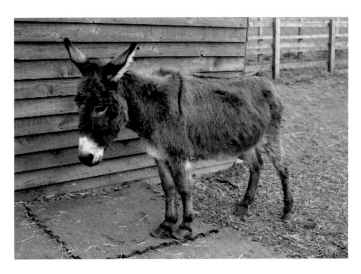

The thick coat of this donkey hid the fact the body condition score was 1. Note also its overgrown hooves and dull demeanour.

CLINICAL EXAMINATION

➜ *See Appendix 1 for a summary chart of the clinical examination.*

In the experience of The Donkey Sanctuary, many older donkeys that owners wish to relinquish into its care have never undergone a dental examination, are not vaccinated, and have either foot or joint pathology, or both.

Owners may recognise that the donkey is behaving differently. It may be lying down more, not lying down as much, has reduced activity, or has changed in demeanour. For example the once bright and alert donkey is now quieter, wandering aimlessly and not interacting with its companions to the same degree. They are, however, likely to put this down to advancing years rather than disease.

As part of a normal examination, the clinician should place particular emphasis on:

* the general demeanour and mobility of the donkey

* body condition score

* assessment of loss of muscle/redistribution of fat

* ease with which joints can be flexed/extended without resultant behavioural signs of pain

* vision.

One of the difficulties of condition scoring old donkeys is that large crests and fat pads may be retained, particularly if calcified, while there is minimal cover, and even muscle wasting, overall.

➜ *See Appendix 3 for a summary chart for body scoring the donkey.*

A test feed is often advisable to ensure that the donkey is prehending, masticating and swallowing effectively.

Feet will still need to be examined, even if arthritis is evident in limb joints, but keeping the foot as close to the ground as possible will minimise the risk of inducing pain and loss of balance in the donkey.

A blood sample for a routine screen should always include an assessment of triglycerides in the donkey where it is presenting as 'dull'.

➜ *See Chapter 7: Hyperlipaemia and the Endocrine System for more information.*

COMMON CONDITIONS

Osteoarthritis is common in both axial and appendicular joints.

The 'stiff donkey' needs to be carefully assessed for joint pain and the owner should be asked to observe if the donkey is able to lie down and get up with ease. The ability to roll should also be assessed, because this is a natural and important behaviour in donkeys. A donkey which never has straw or shavings (or other substrates) adherent to the trunk

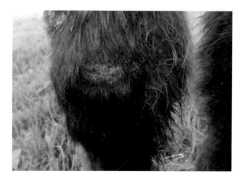

Lesions in the donkey indicating difficulty in lying and/or rising.

or rug may not be lying down at all and this may be because it finds rising difficult – a fearful situation for a prey species. Carpal and hock lesions may be indicative of difficulty in lying and/or rising.

> ⚠ **ALERT**
>
> The farrier should be advised when a donkey suffers from arthritis, because lifting the feet too far off the ground could result in unnecessary pain, consequent resistance behaviour, and a lack of balance.

Reluctance on the part of the donkey to allow anyone to lift its feet may be wrongly attributed to resistant behaviour, but may actually be a result of arthritic pain.

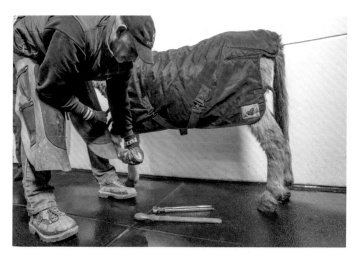

Consider arthritic pain when lifting the foot of the geriatric donkey.

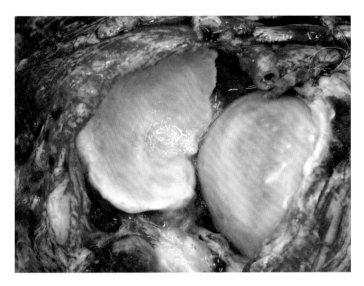

Severe osteoarthritic changes in the hip joint of a donkey that simply presented as 'stiff'. Note significant erosion of cartilage on both femoral head and acetabular surfaces.

➔ *See Chapter 9: The Musculoskeletal System for more information.*

The arthritic donkey may not have the full range of comfortable neck movement and consideration should be given to adjusting the height of food and water containers to allow for this.

'Stiffness' in the donkey usually equates to pain. Continuing stiffness despite analgesia would warrant euthanasia, because arthritic pain is likely to be unremitting.

Analgesics should be prescribed and the response must be closely monitored.

➔ *See Chapter 17: Pharmacology and Therapeutics for more information.*

Laminitis is common in the older donkey and there may well be a legacy of untreated attacks over decades, resulting in unremitting foot pain but only manifesting as short stridedness, a 'pottery' gait, or subtle shifting of weight from limb to limb. Tell-tale laminitic rings may well be present and a dropped and/or thin sole evident.

Some donkeys will not respond reliably to hoof testers; these tend to be the thick-soled mammoth breeds of donkeys.

Radiographs will confirm the extent of pathology and assist the remedial farrier.

The different anatomy of the donkey means that frog supports are contraindicated (unless radiographs indicate otherwise), because the point of frog is behind the fulcrum of the pedal bone.

➜ *See Chapter 9: The Musculoskeletal System for more information about treatment and analgesia, including the use of epoxy resin to form 'false shoes'.*

> ⚠ **ALERT**
>
> **The point of frog is normally behind the fulcrum of the pedal bone in the donkey, and therefore frog supports may be contraindicated.**

The images illustrate significant laminitic change in a 'pottery/stiff' donkey that had never been diagnosed before arrival at The Donkey Sanctuary. This emphasises the concerns regarding the diagnosis of pain related conditions in this stoic animal.

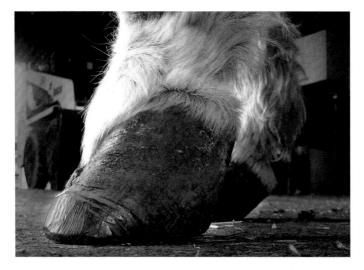

Clear signs of laminitic change with laminitic hoof wall 'rings' diverging towards the overgrown heel.

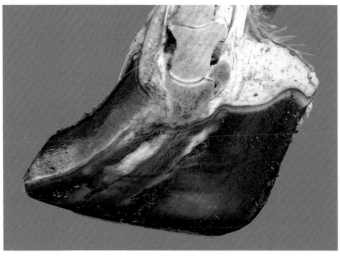

Findings from the post-mortem examinstion show severe degeneration of P3 and a massively overgrown hoof wall.

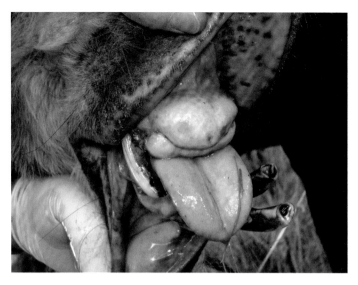

Extensive abnormality of incisors in an aged donkey.

Dental disease, with or without associated sinus disease, occurs frequently in donkeys of all ages but is compounded by time and a lack of professional dental care on a regular basis. It is well recognised that dental pain is one of the most severe sources of pain in horses and ponies, and this is no different for the donkey.

Common abnormalities seen in older donkeys relinquished to The Donkey Sanctuary include periodontal disease, diastemata, malocclusions, dental overgrowths resulting in both hard and soft tissue pathology (eg penetration of opposing bony structures) and tooth loss.

It is important to make a full patient assessment and a treatment plan in order to prevent any unforeseen consequences from treatment.

➔ *See Chapter 2: The Head and Oral Cavity for more information on dental disease.*

Sight impairment may occur as a result of age related cataracts or repeated attacks of uveitis that have gone undiagnosed or untreated.

The Donkey Sanctuary would not consider transportation of a blind donkey for the purpose of rehoming or in any circumstances other than an emergency, and would recommend euthanasia in the home to be the best welfare outcome if the owner is no longer able to keep the donkey.

Pituitary pars intermedia dysfunction (PPID), also known as Cushing's disease is recognized in donkeys.

The thick coat of the donkey can make weight loss/gain and altered fat deposition less obvious.

Hirsuitism and curliness of the coat are less frequently recognized in the

PPID donkey.

High internal and external parasite burdens commonly accompany PPID.

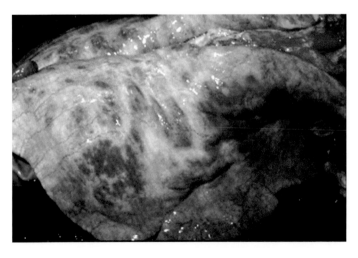 *See Chapter 7: Hyperlipaemia and the Endocrine System for more information.*

Internal parasite related disease is common in donkeys of all ages, no less so in the geriatric. The donkey may never have been wormed or, indeed, may have been 'over' treated, and pasture management may have been lacking. Cyathastominosis may result in colitis and catastrophic loss of proteins or insidious weight loss.

See Chapter 11: Parasitology for more information.

Liver disease may be diagnosed as a result of a combination of analysis of blood samples, ultrasonography/biopsy and clinical signs that include weight loss, dullness and neurological signs.

Respiratory compromise. It is frequently found that pulmonary fibrosis may have gone unnoticed in the non-athletic donkey until dypsnoea is obvious at rest.

Tracheal collapse is not uncommon and is a result of age related degeneration of the tracheal rings and cartilage.

The two conditions can occur together.

Steroids may provide temporary improvement but, with no effective long-term treatment available, the chronic tachypnoiec/dyspnoeic donkey should be euthanased.

See Chapter 4: The Respiratory System for more information.

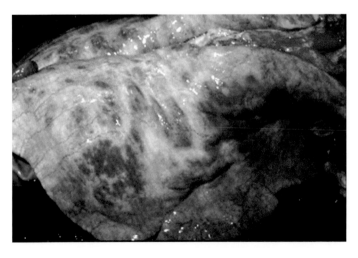

Severe fibrosis of the lungs.

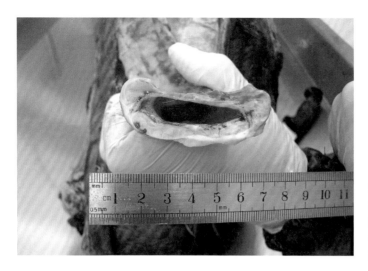

Collapsed trachea revealed at post-mortem examination in a geriatric donkey.

Mental decline. Age related mental decline is not uncommon in donkeys and should be a consideration in any quality of life assessment in the geriatric individual.

Behaviour change, particularly a change in the way companion donkeys interact, may be significant. Lifelong companions may interact less in the face of terminal disease, with the healthier of the two donkeys appearing to abandon its companion.

GERIATRIC MANAGEMENT

Several options are available to ensure that the geriatric donkey has a comfortable life. These will not all be appropriate or even possible for every case. Decisions regarding a suitable management plan should be agreed in discussions with the owner.

- For the older donkey, particularly those with a degree of osteoarthritis, fields should be as flat as possible, because slopes will present a constant challenge and may result in reduced activity.

- Water, feed and shelter should be readily accessible at all times.

- A deep shavings bed is easier to negotiate than straw. Shavings are also recommended for the donkey with dental disease, to reduce the risk of digestive impactions through the inability to process long fibre.

- A stable-safe heat lamp should be advised in temperate/cold climates, and the donkey may require rugging.

- The rugged donkey requires extra vigilance and the owner should be advised to remove the rug daily to check for any lesions.

➔ *See online at **thedonkeysanctuary.org.uk/for-professionals** for information on donkey shaped rugs.*

- Apart from lesions caused by rugging, the owner should be vigilant for any lesions appearing on the carpal and hock joints, which would indicate difficulty in lying or rising.

- Donkeys appear to have an aversion to very cold water, which may result in a reluctance to drink during the cold months. Water with the 'chill' taken off it will be more readily acceptable and may reduce the risk of dehydration and digestive impactions. While thermostatically controlled water-supply systems are now available, it is just as easy and less expensive to add hot water to the bucket/trough on at least a twice-daily basis.

- Dental disease will necessitate a specific diet, usually in the form of a short chop forage. There are now high-fibre, low-calorie short chop products available such that *ad libitum* feeding can be practised, thus satisfying the behavioural need of a trickle feeder. Should the dental disease progress such that only 'gruel' can safely be fed, then quality of life should be discussed with the owner, bearing in mind that a donkey's normal behaviour would be to eat for up to 16 hours in a 24 hour period.

➡ *See Chapter 18: Nutrition for more information.*

- Key to managing the sight impaired donkey is that the environment remains unchanged. Judicious padding of shelter/stable doorways may be appropriate, and mangers and troughs should be checked to ensure they will not cause injury to the donkey. Some donkeys benefit from being fitted with a padded 'bumper' head collar.

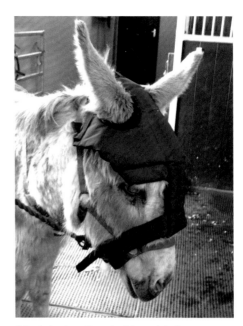

Blind donkey fitted with padded head collar.

ASSESSMENT OF QUALITY OF LIFE

If euthanasia is not immediately indicated or accepted by the owner, it is a valuable exercise to monitor changes or progressive decline by examining and recording specified parameters.

The owner can be given a monitoring sheet to record the health and welfare of their donkey. 'Monitoring your donkey's quality of life' has been produced and used by The Donkey Sanctuary.

➡️ *See Appendix 5 for the template sheet: Monitoring your donkey's quality of life.*

The owner should be advised to complete a sheet on a daily or weekly basis and to discuss the findings with their vet on a regular basis. The parameters included in the sheet give a good indication of the health and, importantly, the welfare of the donkey, and will enable the owner to see any progress or decline and feed the information that they have observed into the assessment record that their vet or other professionals should keep.

It will allow an informed and objective discussion between the owner and the vet or other professionals when the welfare of the donkey is compromised. The assessment record for the quality of life of the donkey will allow a record to be kept of discussions, owner reports and professional or paraprofessional assessment. This will include a defined end point, for example the point at which analgesia is failing to control arthritic pain.

➡️ *See Appendix 6 for the template sheet: Veterinary Record of Assessment for Quality of Life.*

If the quality of life of the individual is poor and treatment options limited by severity of disease or financial considerations, then euthanasia is likely to be the best outcome for the donkey's welfare.

Euthanasia should not be considered a failure, but the last good thing that can be done for the donkey.

It is important to consider the companion animal when a decision has been made to euthanase a donkey. Plans must always be made to address the bereavement that the companion is likely to experience.

➡️ *See Chapter 15: Euthanasia and the Post-Mortem Examination for more information on euthanasia and bereavement management.*

Findings from the Advancing Equine Scientific Excellence (AESE) End of Life project were that vets provide an important role in supporting owners when making the decision to euthanase their donkey at the most appropriate time. Quality of life assessments are often done on an informal basis between the vet and the owner. However these are rarely logged so cannot be referred back to when monitoring decline in chronic conditions. There can also be a discrepancy between an owner's perception of quality of life and what is actually being assessed, so this is an important area of education for owners. Where they were asked, owners requested more information on geriatric care and quality of life assessment.

➔ See **thedonkeysanctuary.org.uk/for-professionals** for more information in the video: Growing Old Gracefully.

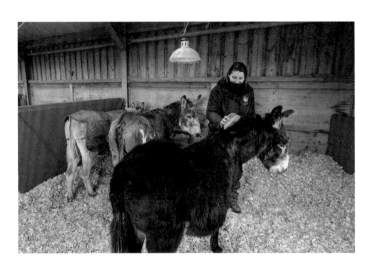

Geriatric donkeys in well bedded pens with bumper pads and a heat lamp.

🐴 MULES AND HINNIES

There is very limited information and evidence available for the mule and therefore nothing to add that is specific to the mule.

ⓘ FURTHER INFORMATION

Factsheets, research and detailed information can be found online at: **thedonkeysanctuary.org.uk/for-professionals**

The video 'Growing Old Gracefully' can be found online at **thedonkeysanctuary.org.uk/for-professionals**

Advancing Equine Scientific Excellence (AESE) End of Life project can be found online at **bef.co.uk/Detail.aspx?page=AESE**

15. EUTHANASIA AND THE POST-MORTEM EXAMINATION

Donkeys are stoic animals. They frequently hide pain and display subtle clinical signs. This must be taken into account when assessing quality of life, an important consideration when deciding on treatment or control of a condition. Unrecognised disease or even recognised conditions, may lead to pain and distress. Unremitting pain, anxiety or chronic discomfort will inevitably impair the donkey's quality of life.

Euthanasia should be considered where the quality of life of a donkey is compromised.

A thorough post-mortem examination is a valuable tool to identify the cause of death, both because clinical signs are often subtle and because there is a need to share information and evidence regarding the health and welfare of donkeys.

QUALITY OF LIFE AND THE DECISION TO EUTHANASE

PREPARING FOR EUTHANASIA

METHODS OF EUTHANASIA

THE COMPANION AND BEREAVEMENT

THE POST-MORTEM EXAMINATION

ANATOMICAL DIFFERENCES

KEY POINTS

- The landmark on the head for humane destruction by shooting is slightly higher in the donkey than in horses and ponies.

- The surviving donkey may be at risk of bereavement associated hyperlipaemia for at least three weeks after the death of its companion.

QUALITY OF LIFE AND THE DECISION TO EUTHANASE

Where the quality of life of the donkey is such that it is either 'having more bad days than good' or is just having bad days, then euthanasia should be carried out without delay.

➡️ *See Chapter 14: The Geriatric Donkey and Quality of Life for more information.*

The assessment and monitoring of quality of life should be an exercise that includes owners, their vet and other professionals. Observation and recording are important elements that allow an informed discussion and provide justification for any advice given.

Templates for owner monitoring sheets and veterinary assessment records are available. These have been used by The Donkey Sanctuary and are recommended for this purpose.

➡️ *See appendix 5 for a template for Monitoring your Donkey's Quality of Life.*

The owner monitoring sheet allows the owner to observe and monitor specific parameters and helps identify any deterioration. This may also help the owner to recognise the need to euthanase their donkey and to reach this decision together with their vet. It should be used to feed into the record sheet with the end-point assessment.

➡️ *See appendix 6 for a template for Veterinary Record of Assessment for Quality of Life.*

The Advancing Equine Scientific Excellence (AESE) UK End of Life project reported that:

Owners rely heavily on their vet for provision of information about quality of life and end of life planning and are happy for their vet to ask them to complete an end of life plan. When asked, owners said they would like information on costs and methods of euthanasia and carcass disposal. This included planning for euthanasia and carcass disposal. Lack of information does result in delays in euthanasia. When asked, owners said they would prefer to get information from direct discussion with their vet. However they would also like to have printed information available from their vet and will use trusted websites such as their veterinary practice to access information.

➲ *See website **bef.co.uk/Detail.aspx?page=AESE** for more information on the AESE End of Life project.*

PREPARING FOR EUTHANASIA

When preparing and planning for euthanasia it is important to consider:

- The bonded companion: donkeys tend to form strong bonds with their companions, and this is an essential consideration when planning for euthanasia. The weeks following euthanasia must also be part of the planning. See the later section on 'The Companion' for more information.

- The use of restraint: many donkeys have not been trained to the head collar and the owner may not be the best person to restrain the donkey at the time of euthanasia.

➜ *See Chapter 1: Behaviour for more information on restraint of the donkey.*

METHODS OF EUTHANASIA

Intravenous injection

Prior sedation may be indicated and may be administered orally or by injection.

However, it is important to note that **xylazine must not be used to sedate prior to the use of secobarbital (somulose)** as violent convulsions may occur.

 See Chapter 16: Sedation, Anaesthesia and Analgesics for more information on sedation.

> ⚠ **ALERT**
>
> The *cutaneous colli* is thicker in donkeys than in horses and ponies and the needle angle needs to be adjusted accordingly for accurate access to the jugular vein.

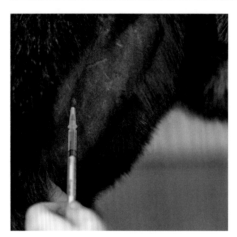 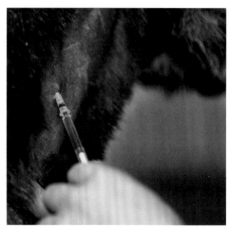

The angle used for intravenous injection in the donkey is typically steeper than in horses and ponies.

> ⓘ **INFORMATION**
>
> **Procedure: Intravenous injection**
>
> - Donkeys may have a thick coat and clipping is advisable to give clear visibility of the vein.
>
> - Donkeys have a prominent *cutaneous colli* muscle which can conceal the middle third of the jugular groove. Therefore the upper third or lower third of the jugular groove is often the best site for injection.
>
> - The angle of needle introduction may need to be adjusted from that in the horse and pony and is typically steeper.

Secobarbital sodium (quinalbarbitone sodium) 400 mg/ml combined with cinchocaine hydrochloride 25mg/ml (Somulose) and used at the standard equine dose (1ml/10kg) is effective in donkeys.

Most donkeys of about 10hh do not weigh more than 200kg so 20mls is normally a suitable dose for a donkey of this size.

Other **barbiturate based drugs** should be used at standard equine doses.

Alternative options are described below.

These should only be employed when there is no alternative and only in the anaesthetised or unconscious donkey:

1. **Tanax (T61)** is a solution with three components (embutramide, mebenzonium iodide and tetracaine hydrochloride) The drug acts by weight of paralysis of respiratory musculature and causes asphyxiation and therefore extreme distress in a conscious animal.

2. **Potassium chloride** (supersaturated) may be injected intravenously or via an intracardiac injection.

3. **Intrathecal lidocaine** will cause cardiac arrest but may take up to 10 minutes. Clip an area over the atlanto-occipital space and use a 16-gauge catheter used for administration of 2% lidocaine hydrochloride at a dosage of 4mg/kg over 30 seconds.

> ⚠ **ALERT**
>
> Tanax, potassium chloride and intrathecal lidocaine must only be used in the anaesthetised or unconscious donkey.

Humane destruction by shooting

It is essential to take account of legislation and best practice, including health and safety considerations, as in horses and ponies.

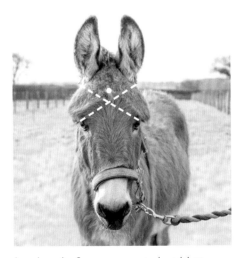

Landmarks for an accurate headshot.

*   The landmark for a head shot is slightly higher than in horses and ponies.

*   The recommended site in the average donkey is 1—2cm above the intersection of two lines drawn between the base of the ear and the contralateral lateral canthus.

Captive Bolt

- **It is important to take account of legislation and best practice, including health and safety considerations, as in horses and ponies.**

- Use of the captive bolt may be effective in skilled hands and it is compulsory to carry out pithing or rapid exsanguination after its use. In a public place both procedures are unacceptable.

THE COMPANION AND BEREAVEMENT

Donkeys tend to form strong bonds with their companions and bereavement management is an important part of planning for euthanasia.

This should be considered in the decision about when and where the euthanasia is carried out.

> ⚠ **ALERT**
>
> The potential distress experienced by a donkey following euthanasia of a companion can lead to bereavement associated hyperlipaemia.

The potential distress to the companion donkey and the subsequent risk of developing hyperlipaemia can be reduced. The following recommendations need to be discussed with the owner and considered on a case by case basis:

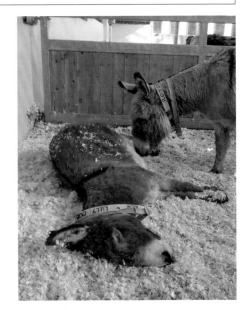

It is important to consider the companion when planning euthanasia.

- The companion donkey should be allowed to 'come to terms' with the death of their companion by leaving the body of the euthanased donkey in an accessible location. This may cause distress to the owner.

- The body should be left with the companion until the companion loses interest. This may take several minutes or several hours.

- The risk of bereavement associated hyperlipaemia remains high for at least three weeks after the loss of a bonded companion, particularly if the bereaved donkey is now living alone.

- It may be advisable to take a blood sample from the surviving donkey to assess triglyceride levels if there is any concern during the period up to three weeks after the event.

- The risk of hyperlipaemia can be reduced by increased interaction on the part of the carer (but not including increased feeding of 'treats') and vigilant monitoring for any dullness or other behavioural change.

- The appetite should be monitored carefully and any sign of a reduction in appetite will require immediate attention.

➔ *See Chapter 7: Hyperlipaemia and the Endocrine System for more information on stimulating appetite.*

- Some owners may be keen to obtain a new donkey immediately but this can be yet another stressor for the surviving donkey. It may be recommended that the introduction of a new companion should be delayed for two to three weeks.

- It may be difficult to source a healthy older donkey but the owner should be advised that the introduction of a young, vigorous donkey to a frail geriatric would not be in the best welfare interests of either.

- Where two bonded donkeys are both frail geriatrics it may be that euthanasia of both is indicated and this would represent a sound welfare outcome. Euthanasia of both would also be indicated if the surviving donkey is blind and has relied upon its companion for guidance.

➔ *See Chapter 1: Behaviour for more information on grief.*

THE POST-MORTEM EXAMINATION

⚠ ALERT

Recognition of signs of illness or pain is often difficult in this stoic animal so information from a post-mortem examination can be valuable.

Information from the post-mortem examination can:

- help detect the reason why treatment has been unsuccessful in some cases

- provide a definitive diagnosis or a differential diagnosis where possible

- provide evidence in legal cases, such as welfare cases

- aid research, for example by identifying and describing new conditions and infectious agents

- contribute to public health by detecting and preventing risks from zoonoses

- provide health protection by identifying contagious, rapidly transmitted infectious disease and enabling advice about the best biosecurity practice

- provide valuable material for educational purposes such as training veterinary students and CPD for veterinary surgeons.

The Donkey Sanctuary would always encourage clinicians to share or publish information gained so that we can expand our evidence based knowledge.

➡ *Email **lab@thedonkeysanctuary.org.uk** to contact our laboratory team for sharing information.*

Post-mortem examination may include weighing the donkey, and should include taking any other measurements, such as girth measurement and body score. The body score is an important tool and is specific to the donkey.

➡ *See appendix 3 for body scoring in the donkey.*

The donkey will often have fibrosed adipose deposits in the crest and dorsally over the ribs, which can persist despite extreme weight loss and emaciation. Body condition score can be judged by assessing the fat cover over the lateral aspects of the ribs. Other condition-scoring landmarks, such as spinous processes, may be altered by post-mortem changes such as rigor. The muscle cover at any body condition score is likely to be less in a geriatric donkey than in a young fit working animal with comparable adipose deposits.

Typically retroperitoneal fat in the ventral abdomen will be several centimetres thick in a donkey of condition score 3 to 4, and as much as 10cm in donkeys of body condition score 5. There will also be considerable retroperitoneal adipose tissue around the kidneys and pelvic viscera.

Assessing the neck crest fat deposits is important in donkeys, because some donkeys retain the fat in the neck crest even after losing weight.

When examining the stomach, inspect the gastric mucosa for ulceration. Most pathology will affect the non-glandular mucosa adjacent to the margo plicatus, the border between glandular and non-glandular parts of the stomach.

The favoured site of tapeworm (*Anoplocephala perfoliata*) attachment in the horse and pony is the ileo-caecal junction, although in donkeys in the UK most tapeworms are found within the caecum at post-mortem examination.

The donkey caecum is similar to that of the horse and pony, but with a shorter, rounder apex. The contents are generally very watery, with small amounts of fibre. Inspection of the mucosal wall will often reveal vacated cysts of the larval stages of the cyathostomins (1mm opaque white circles and semi-spheres). Some paler cysts may contain larvae just visible to the naked eye as tiny black dots. When large numbers of larvae are entering or leaving the mucosa, considerable ulceration and inflammation can occur, resulting in marked oedema. If mucosa without oedema is stripped and examined with a back-light under a dissecting microscope, the larvae can be visualised and counted so that a larval density can be calculated.

The presence of active parasitic arteritis due to *Strongylus vulgarus* is probably quite rare in the UK and other similar countries, due to widespread use of modern anthelmintics. In other environments parasitic arteritis may be more common. Once developed, these lesions of the cranial mesenteric artery do not resolve rapidly.

Despite pre-mortem anorexia, it is not uncommon for the stomach to contain substantial amounts of ingesta. This should be distinguished from gastric impaction, a condition usually associated with chronic hepatic disease in the donkey. In these cases, the stomach will be massively distended, often to the point of rupture, with very heavy dry ingesta.

On opening the larynx and trachea, the cartilages should be examined. Tracheal collapse is common in the donkey, with tracheal rings appearing misshapen, overlapping or flattened. The lumen of the respiratory tree may contain some frothy fluid but should be free of muco-purulent exudates or parasites (*Dictyocaulus arnfieldii*).

In female donkeys the ovaries are located near the kidneys within the caudal abdomen. During anoestrus the ovaries are a little larger than big kidney beans. During the breeding season the ovaries will be the size of quail eggs.

Asymptomatic granulosa cell tumours have not been reported in the donkey, although large, fluid-filled 'cysts' will occasionally be found that can be associated with colic. These are filled with sterile, dark, watery fluid and are likely to be follicles that failed to reach the ovulation fossa (anovulatory follicles). In some cases they can be football-size. Frequently, rupture of small vessels in the anovulatory follicles may lead to haemorrhage and secondary haemoabdomen as a consequence of a ruptured anovulatory follicle.

ANATOMICAL DIFFERENCES

Anatomical differences may be viewed as adaptations to the donkey's natural environment:

- The large ears are useful to receive communication from disparate groups and to aid in heat dissipation.

- The angled epiglottis, narrow nasal meatuses, and expanded.

- nasopharyngeal recess play a role in the production of the characteristic resonant bray of this species, which can carry across many kilometres.

- The bones of the head area are much larger than in a comparably sized pony, with a very powerful jaw capable of grinding lignin-rich plants and shrubs.

- The maxillary sinus is divided into rostral and caudal compartments by a thin, incomplete, bony septum, in contrast to the horse and pony which have a complete bony septum, which allows easier drainage.

- The short neck and protruding manubrium support the heavy skull, leading to an increased thickness of the cutaneous coli muscle.

- The distal punctum of the nasolacrimal duct opens far dorsomedially within the nostril, well placed to avoid blockage with sand.

- The abdomen often appears to be more pendulous than in the horse and pony due to a high-fibre diet, lack of muscle tone, and intra-abdominal fat deposits.

- The sacrum of the horse is a relatively flat bone with five segments. The donkey's sacrum also has five segments, but often the first coccygeal vertebra is fused to the sacrum with occlusion of the sacrococcygeal space.

- The donkey sacrum is curved dorsoventrally, directing the spinal canal ventrally in the caudal segments. The sacral spines point backwards and rapidly decrease in length caudally. The spinal canal slopes backward more steeply, to end at the third coccygeal vertebra. The spinal cord ends at the second sacral vertebral segment, whereas the dural sheath extends back to the first or second coccygeal vertebra.

- The coccygeal vertebrae are much better developed in donkeys than in horses, with the vertebral arches of the first three being complete and each having interarcuate ligaments.

- The first intercoccygeal space in the donkey is narrower than the second space. In horses the spinal cord ends at the junction of the first and second sacral vertebral segments and the dural envelope at the fourth sacral segment. The vertebral arches of the second and third coccygeal vertebrae of horses are incomplete, with an absence of any interarcuate ligaments.

- The upright hooves and typically close limbs are suited for movement in difficult terrain, rather than for speed.

- The vertebral formula for the donkey is C7, T18, L5, S5, Ca 15–17.

- The dorsal top line of the donkey, with its low withers, straight back and smooth, slow paces, has encouraged its use as a pack and draught animal rather than as an athlete of the equine world.

- The ergots of the donkey tend to be more prominent and suggestive of a vestigial foot pad.

- Some male donkeys have teats on their sheath and have proportionately longer reproductive organs than horses.

- The anatomy of the cervix of the female donkey differs from that of the horse and pony, not only in size (being longer than the mare's, and smaller in diameter), but also in the existence of a large protrusion from the cervix into the vagina.

- There are dorsal and ventral folds in the vaginal region that impede passage to the cervix, but they can be relaxed.

Average anatomical measurements of the 'normal' internal organs from a study of 43 UK donkeys (Source: The Donkey Sanctuary):

Body Weight (BW)	Gut		Stomach		Liver	
	Weight (W) (kg)	% BW	W (kg)	% BW	W (kg)	% BW
178.6	44.4	24.6	6.6	3.6	2.8	1.6

Caecum				Large Colon	Small Colon
W (kg)	% BW	Length (L) (cm)	Diameter (D) (cm)	L (cm)	L (cm)
5.9	3.4	79.7	17.6	275.9	111.9

Transverse Colon	Small Intestine	Rectum	Kidneys		Heart	
L (cm)	L (cm)	L (cm)	W (kg)	% BW	W (kg)	% BW
9.8	1110	30	1.2	0.8	1.2	0.7

🐴 MULES AND HINNIES

There is very limited information and evidence available for the mule and therefore nothing to add that is specific to the mule.

ℹ️ FURTHER INFORMATION

Factsheets, research and detailed information can be found online at: **thedonkeysanctuary.org.uk/for-professionals**

The Working Equid Veterinary Manual: **thebrooke.org/for-professionals/ working-equid-veterinary-manual**

King, J.M. *et al* (2014) The Necropsy Book: A Guide for Veterinary Students, Residents, Clinicians, Pathologists, and Biological Researchers, Cornell University.

Buergelt, C. D. and Del Piero, F. (2014) Color Atlas of Equine Pathology, Wiley Blackwell.

Zachary, F.J. (2017) Pathologic Basis of Veterinary Disease, 6th edition, Elsevier.

Aleman, M. et al (2015) Electrophysiologic Study of a Method of Euthanasia Using Intrathecal Lidocaine Hydrochloride Administered during Intravenous Anaesthesia in Horses. *Journal of Veterinary Internal Medicine* 29 (6), 1676—1682.

The Working Equid Veterinary Manual (2013) pp 163—170. Whittett Books Ltd, UK.

16. SEDATION, ANAESTHESIA AND ANALGESIA

Donkeys differ from horses and ponies, with differences in anatomy, physiology and temperament that are important to be aware of when planning sedation, anaesthesia and analgesia. Protocols for donkeys may be based upon those used in horses and ponies, but careful attention must be paid to the different pharmacological and handling requirements as well as the variations necessary for certain procedures. It is also important to note the difficulties in judging the weight of a donkey.

The doses for drugs may be different to those used in horses and ponies because of an altered drug metabolism. Such differences are thought to be a result of the donkey being a desert adapted animal, with differing body fluid compartment distribution and faster oxidative metabolism of many drugs compared to horses and ponies.

Many of the drugs are not authorised for use in the donkey and the use of these drugs must be in accordance with local regulations for prescribing unlicensed medication.

SEDATION

GENERAL ANAESTHESIA

ANALGESIA

REGIONAL ANAESTHESIA

ANAESTHESIA IN FOALS

KEY POINTS

- Estimation of weight requires donkey specific techniques.

- Drug dosages and pharmacokinetics/dynamics are different to those in horses and ponies.

- Endotracheal intubation can be challenging.

- It is not uncommon for donkeys to sneeze subsequent to sedation with alpha-2 agonist drugs.

- There is a high risk of hyperlipaemia associated with the peri-operative period.

- There is a risk of missing underlying disease and/or pain due to the stoic nature of the donkey.

- Donkeys have different baseline physiological parameters.

- Consider donkey specific behaviour traits such as strong bonding with companions and techniques for handling.

SEDATION

Sedation in donkeys for stressful and painful procedures, or prior to anaesthesia, is broadly similar to horses and ponies.

⚠ ALERT

Donkeys have thicker skin and anatomical differences which require an adapted intravenous injection technique.

The common route of sedative administration will be by intravenous injection. Differences in anatomy which make intravenous access more challenging in the donkey are described on the following page.

Sedation can be done 'off the needle', but for prolonged procedures catheterisation is advisable because intravenous injection can be challenging in the donkey and frequent top-ups are often necessary.

ℹ INFORMATION

Procedures: Intravenous injection

- Donkeys may have a thick coat and clipping is advisable to give clear visibility of the vein.

- Donkeys have a thick skin. It is advisable to inject a small quantity of local anaesthetic intradermally and make a small incision in the skin prior to catheter placement.

- A 14 gauge 80mm catheter is suitable for the majority of donkeys.

- Donkeys have a prominent *cutaneous colli* muscle which can conceal the middle third of the jugular groove. Therefore the upper third or lower third of the jugular groove is often the best site for injection.

- The angle of needle introduction may need adjusting from that in the horse and pony and is typically steeper.

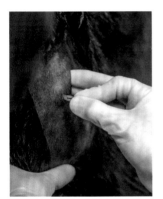 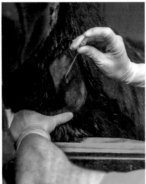 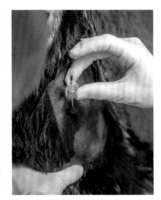

Placing an intravenous catheter.

An initial 'off the needle' administration of sedative may assist catheter placement in less cooperative patients. The use of oral or intramuscular sedation in fractious animals is discussed below.

The dose of sedative agent used will depend on the temperament, age and health status of the donkey, and the anticipated duration and potential pain level of the procedure.

⚠ ALERT

Top-ups of the sedative are often necessary at more frequent intervals than in horses and ponies due to the more rapid drug metabolism.

Note that:

- All of the commercially available alpha-2 agonists can be successfully used in the donkey using standard equine doses. Precise selection is according to availability, personal experience and the procedure being undertaken.

- Sedation top-ups may need to be administered more frequently in donkeys than in horses and ponies, due to differing rates of drug metabolism.

- Typically the alpha-2 agonists will be combined with an opioid and data sheets must be checked to calculate suitable dosing regimes.

- Local anaesthetic nerve blocks should always be considered when appropriate.

Constant-rate infusions may be advisable for lengthier procedures. Suitable combinations replicate those used in horses and ponies. The clinician is advised to consult standard equine texts and data sheets.

Note that **the normal equine dosing interval may need to be shortened in order to maintain adequate sedation, particularly in fractious individuals,** and the drip rate should be adjusted to effect.

Different routes of administration

There will be occasions when it may be preferable to administer sedatives by the intramuscular or oral route. Examples include sedation of mules, or where there is prior knowledge of a problem in handling a donkey. It is preferable to sedate the donkey before it becomes stressed or experiences fear, and thus improve levels of sedation and reduce long term issues with needle sensitisation.

Options for sedating a donkey are similar to those for nervous or fractious horses and ponies. Clinicians may choose to supply an owner with oral sedative for use prior to their arrival. The Donkey Sanctuary uses oral detomidine gel at standard equine doses.

GENERAL ANAESTHESIA

Pre-anaesthetic preparation

Before planning a general anaesthetic consider whether a standing procedure is a realistic alternative, especially if a donkey is in poor health or geriatric.

It is important to consider the different behaviours and temperaments of the donkey when planning anaesthesia. Be aware that:

- Donkeys may be less used to regular handling than horses and ponies.

- It is essential to have plenty of patience and maintain a calm demeanour.

- A well fitting head collar, supplemented with an arm around the neck and/or a hand over the dorsal nose surface, can provide good restraint.

➡ *See Chapter 1: Behaviour for more information on restraint.*

⚠ **ALERT**

Donkeys are often strongly bonded to their companion.

It is important to consider the strong bond between donkeys when planning anaesthesia or indeed any procedure:

- It is essential that the companion accompanies and remains with the patient until as close to induction as possible.

- If the companion is unsettled or anxious, eg during catheter placement of the patient, it can be useful to separate the donkeys so that they can still maintain eye and muzzle contact over an appropriate gate or stable door.

- Note that while the patient is undergoing anaesthesia the companion may become very stressed at being separated. Initial distraction with attention and food treats can help. Severe cases may require sedation.

- Where there is a known problem, the companion animal can be given an oral sedative such as detomidine gel about 30 minutes before the procedure.

- Where a foal is present there is a high risk of stress to both mare and foal. Donkey foals may require sedation while separated from an anaesthetised mare. The Donkey Sanctuary has used xylazine or detomidine at standard equine foal doses.

Failure to appreciate the significance of companion bonds can induce significant stress and a variable reaction to sedation or anaesthesia.

⚠ **ALERT**

Stress increases the risk of hyperlipaemia.

Be aware of the risks of hyperlipaemia peri-operatively. Particular risk factors are stress due to separation from bonded companions, underlying pain and disease, and pre-anaesthetic starvation.

➜ *See Chapter 7: Hyperlipaemia and Endocrine diseases for more information.*

The Donkey Sanctuary does not recommend prolonged periods of starvation prior to a standard elective anaesthetic and will withhold hard feed and hay overnight, but allow access to straw or grazing until the morning of the operation.

Suckling foals should not be starved.

⚠ **ALERT**

There is a high risk that any underlying disease or pain will be missed because of the stoical temperament of the donkey.

A thorough pre-operative examination is paramount on the day to ascertain the health status of the animal and to obtain baseline physiological parameters.

Remember that the physiological parameters of the donkey differ from those of horses and ponies.

ⓘ **INFORMATION**

Adult donkey physiological parameters

- **Temperature:** 36.5—37.8°C

- **Pulse:** 36—52 beats/minute

- **Respiration:** normally 20 breaths/minute but with a range of 12—28 breaths/minute

Bear in mind that:

- Because of the stoical nature of the donkey, there is a high risk that any disease or painful conditions may be easily missed. The clinician will need to make a judgement on the benefits of pre-anaesthetic blood tests. **Donkey specific reference ranges for biochemistry and haematology must be used for evaluation.**

➜ *See Appendix 4 for the Parameters: Biochemistry and Haematology.*

- Because donkeys are not often kept as athletic individuals, subtle signs of disease may be masked and easily missed. Pay particular attention to any evidence of underlying respiratory disease or subtle lameness.

- Although donkeys may not display overt signs of pain, perioperative analgesia is essential for a smooth anaesthetic and the ongoing well-being of the patient.

Accurate weight estimation is necessary for calculation of anaesthetic drug dosages.

The difficulty in calculating a donkey's weight in the field situation is possibly the biggest cause of poor levels of sedation and anaesthesia.

⚠ **ALERT**

Horse and pony weigh tapes are not suitable for estimating the weight of donkeys.

The Donkey Sanctuary weigh nomogram is available for weight estimation.

➡ *See Appendix 2 for The Donkey Sanctuary Weight Estimator.*

A weigh tape has been developed specifically for the donkey. This is suitable for estimating the weight of a donkey whilst horse and pony weigh tapes are not.

➡ *See online at **www.donkeyweightape.com** for a donkey specific weigh tape.*

Very few drugs are licensed for use in the donkey. The clinician should be aware of the legal requirements of the country in which they are working with regard to prescribing.

For example, currently in the UK, unlicensed medication can be prescribed under the Cascade. The owner must be informed that the medication is unlicensed, the medication must be recorded in the passport, and section ix must be signed to confirm that the animal is not intended for human consumption, if this is to be the case.

In the interests of maintaining hygiene it is advisable to groom donkeys prior to induction.

It is advisable to have a crash kit available for emergencies. Suggested dosages of such drugs are currently the same as in horses and ponies.

Induction

Donkeys that are not used to handling will need plenty of patience. It is essential that the donkey is wearing a head collar for induction and is held by an experienced handler.

➡ *See Chapter 1: Behaviour for more information on restraint.*

The donkey's mouth should have been flushed prior to induction.

While donkeys lack the bulk of horses, they can still go down quickly and with force. Induction should be carried out in a well-padded environment.

The placement of an intravenous catheter for administration of anaesthetic drugs is strongly recommended. In fractious donkeys, consider giving a small volume of the calculated alpha-2 'off the needle' to facilitate catheter placement. The remainder of the alpha-2 dose can then be given once the catheter is secured.

Anatomical differences in the donkey mean that modified intravenous techniques may be required.

➡ *See the previous section on sedation for more information.*

Standard equine dosages are used for initial anaesthetic induction doses in donkeys.

> ⚠ **ALERT**
>
> A heightened fight or flight response/increased adrenaline as a result of being in an unfamiliar situation may increase the volume of sedative required to achieve a smooth induction.

🖊 **DRUGS**

A typical theatre induction protocol from The Donkey Sanctuary		
Pre-anaesthetic medications	Prophylactic antimicrobials if indicated	Dose as per data sheet for selected antimicrobial. We recommend timing the dose to ensure administration within 60 minutes of first incision
	ACP	0.03mg/kg bwt i.v. or i.m. 30—60 minutes prior to induction
	NSAID	eg Flunixin meglumine 1.1mg/kg bwt i.v.
	Alpha-2 agonist	eg detomidine 0.02mg/kg bwt i.v.
	Opioid	eg butorphanol 0.02mg/kg bwt i.v.
Induction	Ketamine	2.2—2.8mg/kg bwt i.v.
	Diazepam	0.1mg/kg bwt i.v. (note higher than in horses and ponies)

Note that:

* The clinician should select the alpha-2 agonist and opioid according to their own preference and experience and the procedure being performed. Butorphanol, buprenorphine and morphine have all been used at standard equine doses. It is essential to verify any choices using

data sheets.

- The dose of ketamine may vary between clinicians and the nature of the donkey. Typically 2.5mg/kg bwt i.v. of ketamine post adequate sedation gives a smooth induction.

Maintenance of anaesthesia

Anaesthesia may be maintained with inhalation or injectable agents.

Inhalation anaesthesia

> ⚠ **ALERT**
>
> Endotracheal intubation can be challenging.

If planning inhalational anaesthesia be aware of the potential difficulties when performing endotracheal intubation:

- The nasopharyngeal airway is short, constricted in the middle, and flared dorsally and ventrally.

- The nasopharyngeal recess (a diverticulum of the pharyngeal mucosa lying between the guttural pouches) is enlarged into a pouch 2—3cm wide and 4—6cm long (in the horse this is 2.5cm long).

- The epiglottis is short and more pointed and the laryngeal opening tilted more caudally.

- The nasal passages are narrower relative to head size compared with horses and ponies.

- The average 180kg donkey requires an endotracheal tube of 16mm internal diameter; if possible, have a range of 14—18mm tubes available.

- Endoscopy may assist laryngeal visualisation.

- Donkeys weighing less than 150kg may need a small animal circuit, because a large animal circuit with excess dead space results in a risk of dyspnoea and hypoxia.

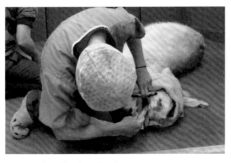 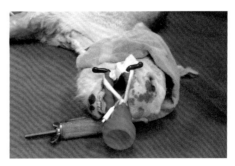

Intubation in the donkey.

Vaporiser setting can be minimised by appropriate use of local anaesthetics and injectable anaesthetic agents.

No donkey specific differences in minimum alveolar concentrations of volatile agents have been noted.

Injectable anaesthesia

> ⚠ **ALERT**
>
> Injectable anaesthetics may need more frequent top-ups due to the more rapid drug metabolism in donkeys.

If injectable agents are used for maintenance of anaesthesia, top-ups may be required more frequently than in horses and ponies due to the shorter half-life of these drugs in donkeys.

Miniature donkeys may require even shorter top-up intervals.

At The Donkey Sanctuary ketamine is commonly used for maintenance as in the table below.

> ✐ **DRUGS**
>
> **Maintenance of anaesthesia using ketamine**
>
> 1/3 of the induction dose of ketamine may be administered approximately every 10 minutes.
>
> Additional topping-up of the alpha-2 agonist, at intervals appropriate to the initial agent given, will provide sedation and may lessen the total volume of ketamine required. As a guide, top up with 1/3—1/2 initial induction dose of alpha-2:
>
> * after 15 minutes if xylazine is used
>
> * after 30 minutes if detomidine used
>
> * after 60 minutes if romifidine is used.

Note that:

* The 'triple drip' combination of guaiphenesin, ketamine and xylazine has also been used for induction and maintenance of anaesthesia in donkeys. A smaller volume of guaiphenesin is needed to induce recumbency in donkeys. Higher amounts of ketamine may be needed in these combinations.

* Guaiphenesin is irritating to perivascular tissues so the catheter should be thoroughly flushed with saline before removal.

As in horses and ponies, there are many recipes. An example used at The Donkey Sanctuary for maintenance of anaesthesia is given below. This may also be used for induction after an alpha-2 pre-medication.

✏ DRUGS

Triple drip recipe used at The Donkey Sanctuary

Donkey triple drip IV at 1—2ml/kg bwt/hr

Rates are approximate and will need adjusting to effect. Donkeys may need smaller volumes of mixture than horses and ponies to maintain anaesthesia.

To make the mixture:

- 300ml 0.9% saline (remove 200ml from a 500ml bag of 0.9% saline and add the other drugs to the remaining 300ml)

- 225ml 10% guaiphenesin

- 225mg xylazine (eg 2.25ml of 100mg/ml (10%) xylazine solution)

- 900mg ketamine (eg 9ml of 100mg/ml (10%) ketamine solution)

N.B. In horses, the lethal dose of guiaphenesin is approximately 300mg/kg. The Donkey Sanctuary does not have proven data confirming the lethal dose in donkeys. Therefore, we currently extrapolate from the lethal dose in horses and are mindful of the knowledge that smaller volumes of guaiphenesin induce recumbency in donkeys.

Avoid dosages greater than 150mg/kg **(1.5ml/kg of guaiphenesin 10% - 270ml for a 180kg donkey)** as cardiovascular and respiratory depression may occur at these high dosages.

TIP: Calculate the toxic dose prior to beginning anaesthesia.

It is not advised to use triple drip for lengthy procedures because the toxic dose of guaiphenesin is liable to be reached.

Triple drip must be used on the day and does not store.

Monitoring Anaesthesia

Monitoring anaesthesia follows the same principles as for horses and ponies. Eye position, pulse, respiratory rate, blood pressure and muscle tension can all be used as indicators of anaesthetic depth.

⚠ ALERT

Judging depth of anaesthesia based on eye position, pulse, respiratory rate, blood pressure and muscle tension may be less predictable in donkeys than horses and ponies.

Note that:

- Monitor trends in parameters over time so that sudden changes become obvious.

- Respiratory rate tends to be higher than in horses and ponies.

- Trends in arterial blood pressure are particularly helpful; be alert to any sudden increases that can accompany a lightening of depth.

- The auricular artery has been used for direct measurement of arterial blood pressure. The facial artery has also been used, or measure indirectly via a cuff.

- Standard machines recording ECG traces, pulse oximetry and capnography can be valuable additional monitoring resources.

- Donkeys usually breathe spontaneously while under general anaesthesia and are less likely to require the use of a ventilator than horses and ponies. It is possible to provide adequate ventilation manually where assistance is needed and a ventilator is not available. Aim for 8—10 breaths/minute, adjusting as necessary if indicated by monitoring.

- Donkeys may breath hold if the plane of anaesthesia is too light.

Be aware that the braying of a patient's companion may lighten depth of anaesthesia. Methods to alleviate this include distracting or sedating the companion as previously described, and placing cotton wool in the patient's ears.

Although myopathies and neuropathies occur less frequently in donkeys undergoing general anaesthesia, appropriate positioning is recommended with padding of trunk and limbs, and fluid therapy as necessary to maintain blood pressure.

Note that perioperative fluid therapy follows the same guidelines as for horses and ponies.

Anaesthesia in the field

It will often be appropriate, or even necessary, to carry out anaesthesia in the field.

While donkeys lack the sheer bulk of horses, they can still go down quickly and with force. Induction should be carried out with care and not on a hard surface.

For anaesthesia in the field it is advisable to take appropriate sized endotracheal tubes and a portable oxygen supply.

The theatre induction protocols described above may also be used where induction is to be carried out in the field. Fractious or feral donkeys may require higher doses. The data sheets should always be consulted, particularly if using variations on suggested protocols.

→ *See online at **thebrooke.org/for-professionals/working-equid-veterinary-manual**: The Working Equid Manual for suitable alternatives where resources are limited or drugs are not available.*

Triple drip recipes can also be used for field surgery but should be approached with caution by the less experienced clinician. Clinicians are advised to familiarise themselves with guaiphenesin anaesthesia using standard equine anaesthesia texts. With triple drip, signs of an appropriate plane of surgical anaesthesia can differ from those seen with inhalational anaesthesia or ketamine top-ups alone.

Regular monitoring of the donkey and recording of vital parameters by trained personnel can be a vital aid to ensuring smooth and safe anaesthesia.

Recovery

The donkey is usually calmer in recovery than horses and ponies and rarely requires sedation.

The donkey will typically delay standing until it is ready and assistance is rarely required, although occasionally a tail pull may be necessary.

There are always exceptions to the rule, so ensure that the donkey is observed until standing.

It is important to ensure analgesia is adequate for the whole post-operative period as the donkey will not always show visible signs of pain.

The owner should be briefed to monitor the donkey closely for any changes in appetite or demeanour over the 2—3 days following the procedure.

ANALGESIA

> ⚠ **ALERT**
>
> Close monitoring and good control of pain during and after surgery is essential.

> ⓘ **INFORMATION**
>
> **Perioperative analgesia in the donkey**
>
> Flunixin 1.1mg/kg **BID** is the first line perioperative choice at The Donkey Sanctuary and may be given for 3—5 days.
>
> Be aware that extended use of flunixin meglumine may mask signs of colic or other painful conditions that may be developing.
>
> Phenylbutazone 2.2mg/kg BID may be used for ongoing analgesia if needed. (Use TID in miniature donkeys).

Flunixin and Phenylbutazone must be prescribed for twice daily (bid) administration in donkeys.

The use of meloxicam is not currently advised in donkeys as it appears to be metabolised too quickly to have any lasting efficacy.

Firocoxib has been used successfully but has not been tried at The Donkey Sanctuary so we do not yet have any data on suitable dosages.

Other analgesics, including ketamine, lidocaine and opioids, have all been used at The Donkey Sanctuary using dosages extrapolated from equine formularies.

REGIONAL ANAESTHESIA

Nerve blocks may be indicated to assist in lameness evaluation, facilitate surgery of the head or distal limb, or for dental procedures.

Local anaesthesia can also provide an invaluable adjunct when performing procedures under general anaesthesia or standing surgery.

The same standard local anaesthetic and regional nerve-blocking techniques used in horses and ponies can be employed. Doses of local anaesthetic may be reduced to reflect the smaller size of the donkey.

Epidurals

When carrying out epidurals be aware that the spinal cord terminates at the level of sacral 2, while the dura may extend to the level of coccygeal 1—2.

Donkeys typically have less musculature over the rump and tail head than horses and ponies, consequently the angle of needle introduction is shallower than in horses and ponies. **Direct the needle at an angle of approximately 30° from the horizontal plane.**

In donkeys it is the **second intercoccygeal space** that is wider and most accessible for needle puncture.

Drugs suitable for epidural administration are as in horses and ponies, using volumes at the lower end of the dose range.

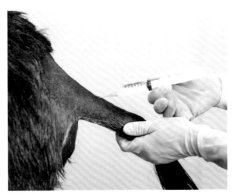 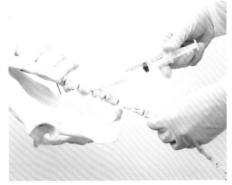

Images showing the location and angle of needle introduction for the epidural.

ANAESTHESIA IN FOALS

Donkey foal anaesthesia follows the same general principles as for other equine foals. Due to the small size of donkey foals, a small animal circuit may be used.

The monitoring and maintenance of body temperature and blood glucose are of particular importance in young foals, especially during prolonged periods of anaesthesia.

There is a high risk of stress to both mare and foal when either one is to be anaesthetised or undergo any procedure. Donkey foals often require sedation during separation from an anaesthetised mare.

 See Chapter 13: The Care of the Foal for more information.

🐴 MULES AND HINNIES

- **Unhandled and fractious mules present a significant health and safety challenge.** Consider the use of personal protective equipment such as a hard hat and body protectors. Dart guns, a chute or appropriate sized stocks may need to be employed.

- Depending on the temperament of the mule and procedure to be performed, **drug dosages may need to be increased by 30—50% above that given for donkeys.**

- When treating fractious mules, which render initial intravenous access dangerous, intramuscular combinations such as equine 'Magic Mix' may provide a safer initial sedative route. This can then be topped up intravenously as necessary.

- The use of oral detomidine gel at standard equine doses has also been effective in providing initial sedation in difficult donkeys. Mules will likely need higher initial doses.

💉 DRUGS

Equine 'Magic Mix' for mules and hinnies

- Detomidine 0.02mg/kg bwt

- ACP 0.03mg/kg bwt

- Butorphanol 0.05mg/kg bwt

- Mix in the same syringe and administer i/m, 1ml of mixture/100kg bwt. Leave unstimulated for 30 minutes.

ℹ️ FURTHER INFORMATION

Factsheets, research and detailed information can be found online at: *thedonkeysanctuary.org.uk/for-professionals*

Matthews, N. and van Loon, J.P.A.M. (2013) Review Article: Anaesthesia and Analgesia of the Donkey and the Mule. *Equine Veterinary Education* 25 (1) 47—51.

Dugdale, A. (2010) Veterinary Anaesthesia, pp 277—278. Wiley-Blackwell, Chichester.

Taylor, E.V., Baetge , C.L., Matthews, N.S., Taylor, T.S. and Barling, K.S. (2008). Guaifenesin-Ketamine-Xylazine Infusions to Provide Anesthesia in Donkeys. *Journal of Equine Veterinary Science* 28 (5) 295—300.

17. PHARMACOLOGY AND THERAPEUTICS

Few veterinary products have market authorisation for use in the donkey. Although preparations designed for horses and ponies are often used for donkeys, there are recorded differences between these species in the pharmacokinetics of certain drugs. An understanding of these differences can enable the practitioner to make appropriate therapeutic decisions to achieve maximum efficacy of medication and reduce the risk of toxicity.

Medicines are included in this chapter only where it has been recorded that there is a notable difference between donkeys and the horse and pony.

Clinicians are advised that they must consult current equine formularies and datasheets. Owners should be informed accordingly and it is imperative that the appropriate national legislation is adhered to.

While we have made every effort to ensure that the content of this chapter is currently accurate, we accept no liability for any loss, damage or expenses arising as a result of relying solely on the information contained within the formulary in this book.

It can be difficult to estimate the weight of a donkey and therefore determine effective dosing regimes. A donkey specific nomogram or a donkey specific weigh tape should be used to estimate weight.

PHARMACOLOGICAL DIFFERENCES OF THE DONKEY

PRESCRIBING FOR THE DONKEY

ADMINISTRATION OF DRUGS AND WEIGHT ESTIMATION

DONKEY SPECIFIC DRUG DOSAGES

KEY POINTS

- Estimating the weight of donkeys is acknowledged to be difficult. A donkey specific nomogram is advised to improve accurate dosing of medication.

- Pharmacokinetics of drugs for donkeys are often different to that for horses and ponies. The clinician is advised to check donkey specific dosage.

- Most drugs are not licensed for use in the donkey. Local legal requirements for prescribing unlicensed medication must be strictly followed.

PHARMACOLOGICAL DIFFERENCES OF THE DONKEY

The donkey's semi arid environment is one of low value forage and limited water supply. The donkey has been reported to tolerate dehydration more effectively than the horse and pony, efficiently recycling water from the large colon and having a lower urine output, even when water is readily available. The donkey has a longer gut transit time. This is one factor leading to an increased feed efficiency and could have an effect on drug absorption. These environmental adaptations may be relevant to the differences in pharmokinetics noted between the donkey and the horse and pony. In addition, there are variations within the species.

For example:

- Miniature donkeys metabolise phenylbutazone at a faster rate than standard donkeys, and therefore require more frequent dosing.

- Mammoth asses have a smaller volume of distribution of gentamicin than standard donkeys.

Hepatic metabolism is often faster in the donkey, with the volume of distribution lower, the clearance rate higher and the half-life shorter than in the horse and pony. In such cases shorter dosing intervals are generally advised rather than larger doses. However, there are important exceptions to this.

⚠ **ALERT**

Where metabolism of a drug is faster in the donkey than in the horse or pony, it is advisable to use shorter dosing intervals rather than larger doses.

In drugs with higher bioavailability and smaller volume of distribution, such as guaiphenesin, there is a higher likelihood of reaching toxic doses in donkeys if the weight is unknown or inappropriate drug doses are used.

PRESCRIBING FOR THE DONKEY

Very few drugs are licensed for use in the donkey. The clinician should be aware of the legal requirements of the country in which they are working with regard to prescribing.

For example, currently in the UK, unlicensed medication can be prescribed under the Cascade.

 *See online at **www.gov.uk/guidance/the-cascade-prescribing-unauthorised-medicines***

The owner must be informed that the medication is unlicensed, the medication must be recorded in the passport, and section ix must be signed to confirm that the animal is not intended for human consumption, if this is to be the case.

ADMINISTRATION OF DRUGS AND WEIGHT ESTIMATION

In order to prescribe safe and effective drug doses, the donkey should have an accurate weight estimated. If no scales are available, the donkey specific weight estimator can be used to estimate the weight of the donkey. A line can be drawn on the nomogram from the heart girth measurement to the height of the donkey, and a weight estimated from these two measurements:

- The heart girth measurement is the circumference of the donkey's thorax just caudal to the elbows, measured in cm.

- Height is measured to the withers in cm.

- Weight is estimated in kg.

➡ *See Appendix 2 for the donkey weight estimator and for a table of weights for donkeys under two years old.*

⚠ **ALERT**

Horse and pony weigh tapes are not appropriate for donkeys.

Intravenous (IV) administration

Differences in anatomy which make intravenous access more challenging in the donkey are described in the box below.

Intravenous catheterisation may be appropriate for repeated medication.

ℹ **INFORMATION**

Procedure: intravenous injection

- Donkeys have a thick coat and clipping is advisable to give clear visibility of the vein.

- Donkeys have thicker skin so placing an intradermal local anaesthetic bleb and nicking the skin, with a scalpel blade prior to catheter placement is advised.

- A 14 gauge 80 mm catheter is suitable for the majority of donkeys, but this is subject to individual preference.

- Donkeys have a prominent cutaneous colli muscle which can conceal the middle third of the jugular groove. Therefore the upper third or lower third of the jugular groove is the best site for injection.

- The angle of needle introduction may need adjusting from that in the horse and pony, and is typically steeper.

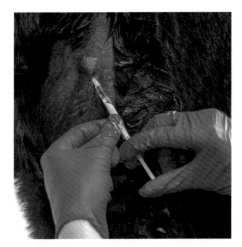
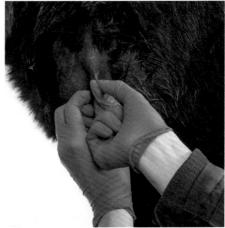
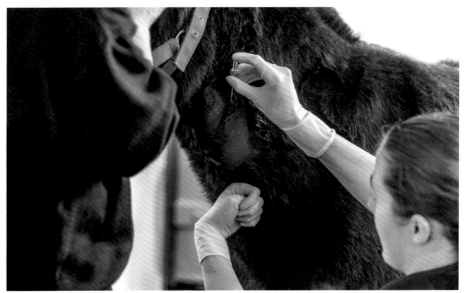

Placing an intravenous catheter.

Intramuscular (IM) administration

Intramuscular injections can be given in the gluteal and neck musculature using the same landmarks as in the horse. However, the pectorals typically have a low muscle mass in the donkey and may not be suitable.

Oral administration

Oral medication can be hidden in feed or more easily administered in jam sandwiches or confectionary.

Epidural

Epidural anaesthesia in the donkey is performed at the second inter-coccygeal space, advancing the needle at an angle of 30 degrees to the horizontal rather than a 45 degree angle at the first inter-coccygeal space as is used in the horse and pony.

➡ *See Chapter 16: Sedation, Anaesthesia and Analgesia for more information.*

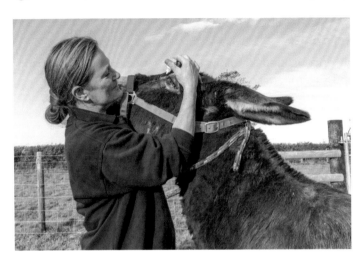

Administering eye ointment.

DONKEY SPECIFIC DRUG DOSAGES

High quality evidence for appropriate drug regimes in donkeys is not available for many of the commonly used medications.

The following table summarises specific differences and identifies drugs that are contra-indicated in the donkey. For all other medications equine datasheets and current formularies should be consulted. Drug company veterinary advisers may also be a source of useful advice.

A note on antimicrobials

Clinicians are strongly encouraged to follow best practice when considering the use of antimicrobials to minimise the risk of promoting resistance.

➡️ *See online toolkit at **beva.org.uk/protectme** for advice on responsible use of antimicrobials.*

Drugs with donkey specific key points

Name of drug	Dose	Route	Comments for use in the donkey
Carprofen	0.7—1.3mg/kg q24hrs	IV PO	Give IV as a single dose. Metabolised more slowly in donkeys.
Etorphine			MUST NEVER BE USED IN THE DONKEY.
Ketamine	2.2—2.8mg/kg bwt	IV	Cleared more rapidly in donkeys, especially miniature donkeys. More frequent top-ups required for TIVA.
Meloxicam	0.6mg/kg	IV	Not advised for use in donkeys – very short half-life.
Phenylbutazone	2.2mg/kg— 4.4mg/kg q12hr in standard, q8hr in miniatures	IV	More rapid clearance than in horses. Administer twice daily to donkeys and three times daily to miniature donkeys.
Flunixin	1.1mg/kg q12hrs	IV	
Fentanyl			Larger dose patch on mg/kg basis required to achieve comparable plasma levels of fentanyl; analgesic levels achieved more rapidly; more frequent patch changes required. Accurate dose rates not confirmed.
Tramadol		PO	Poor oral bioavailability (reported as 11.7%). Not recommended for use in donkeys.
Gentamicin	6.6mg/kg SID	IV	Care in mammoth asses: volume of distribution is lower so take care to avoid toxicity. A lower dose should be used in hypovolaemic animals but a shorter dosing interval may be required to keep levels above MIC.

Oxytetracycline	5-10mg/kg q12—24 hrs	Slow IV	Shorter elimination half-life. Dosing interval should be half that recommended for horses. More data required.
Na Penicillin G	20,000IU/kg IV q4—6hrs	IV	Shorter dosing intervals required in donkeys for beta-lactam antibiotics, more comparative studies required.
Trimethoprim sulphamethoxazole	30 mg/kg q12hrs	PO	Volume of distribution and elimination rate of trimethoprim differs to that of sulphonamides, therefore ratio may not be optimal for donkeys.
Danofloxacin			Does not achieve effective plasma concentrations in donkeys at 1.25mg/kg.
Marbofloxacin	0.33—2.6mg/kg q24hrs	Slow IV	Slower elimination in donkeys. 0.33mg/kg for Enterobacteriaceae sp, 2.6mg/kg Staphylococcus aureus.
Norfloxacin			Not suitable for use in donkeys: IV administration at 10mg/kg has induced seizures, IM has caused local swelling, and oral administration has low availability.
Buprenorphine	5-10µg/kg q8hrs	IV	
Detomidine	0.01—0.04mg/kg 0.04—0.08mg/kg 0.04mg/kg	IV IM Oral gel	Donkeys may require larger doses to achieve adequate sedation. IM dose 1.5—2x IV dose. Maximal effects in quiet, unstimulating environment after injection.
Firocoxib		PO	Good oral bioavailability, shorter half-life than in horses and ponies. More research needed to determine optimum dosing interval.
Dexamethasone	0.05—0.2mg/kg q24hrs	IV, IM or PO	Contraindicated in hyperlipaemic animals.
Guaifenesin	To effect ~50—110mg/kg needed for induction	IV	Metabolised more rapidly in donkeys than horses and ponies but donkeys show greater sensitivity. For a donkey specific 'triple drip' recipe see Chapter 16: Sedation, Anaesthesia and Analgesics.
Heparin sodium	100—200IU/kg q8—12hrs	IV	May be used in hyperlipaemia. Check clotting factors before initiating treatment.
Imidocarb diproprionate	2mg/kg q24hrs for babesia caballi. 4mg/kg q3 days for 4 treatments for babesia equi.	IM IM	DO NOT USE IMIDOCARB DIHYDROCHLORIDE IN DONKEYS. Take care with imidocarb diproprionate as it can cause muscle necrosis, central nervous signs and death at higher doses.

🐴 MULES AND HINNIES

There is very limited information and evidence available for the mule and therefore nothing to add that is specific to the mule.

ℹ️ FURTHER INFORMATION

Factsheets, research and detailed information can be found online at: **thedonkeysanctuary.org.uk/for-professionals**

The Working Equid Veterinary Manual: **thebrooke.org/for-professionals/working-equid-veterinary-manual**

Grosenbaugh, D.A., Reinemeyer, C.R. and Figueiredo, M.D. (2011) Pharmacology and therapeutics in donkeys. *Equine Veterinary Education*, 23 (10) pp523—530.

Lizarraga, I., Sumano, H. and Brumbaugh, G.W. (2004) Pharmacological and pharmacokinetic differences between donkeys and horses. *Equine Veterinary Education.* 16 (2) pp102—112.

Bertone, J.J. and Horspool, L.J. (2004) Equine Clinical Pharmacology. Saunders.

18. NUTRITION

Donkeys have evolved to thrive on highly fibrous, poor quality foodstuffs and have evolved as browsers as well as grazers. As a result they have different nutrient requirements, with significantly lower energy and protein needs than horses and ponies. Dietary management of the donkey is essential to avoid health issues and should be seen as the foundation of a healthy animal.

NUTRITIONAL REQUIREMENTS

THE NORMAL DIET

MONITORING THE DIET

FEEDING FOR COMMON CONDITIONS

FEEDING IN PREGNANCY

KEY POINTS

- A diet based on fibrous forages and limited grazing is usually sufficient for the majority of sedentary donkeys kept as companion animals.

- Working donkeys should be provided with a diet based on fibre, which may include conserved forages such as straws and grazing. Their diet may be supplemented with oils, high quality fibres and limited cereal by-products.

- Donkeys have efficient digestion and have lower energy requirements than horses and ponies of a similar size.

- Donkeys may 'sham eat'; the animal appears to mouth and swallow food or may simply nudge it but does not eat it. Such behaviour is often a sign of a serious illness.

- Body scoring is different for donkeys and protocols used in horses and ponies are not suitable.

The domestic donkey is descended from African wild asses that evolved to live in semi-arid environments with only poor quality, sparse vegetation. To increase their potential source of food, donkeys have evolved to be browsers as well as grazers, with woody shrubs and trees being potential food sources when grasses and other low vegetation are not abundant. Donkeys are trickle feeders; wild donkeys access suitable and sufficient feedstuffs by spending many hours (14—18 hours a day) foraging, and will travel many kilometres to search out the choicest feedstuffs.

Donkeys are highly efficient at digesting poor nutritional quality fibre. They possess a superior digestive efficiency compared to horses and ponies when digesting highly fibrous forages such as straw. These adaptations may be beneficial for working donkeys and allow them to thrive on fibre sources which would be inadequate for horses and ponies managed in the same way.

However, this adaptation to survive on a poorer quality feed can lead to obesity in companion donkeys when they are mistakenly treated in the same way as horses and ponies. Obesity is also likely where donkeys are kept together with horses or ponies and are not fed and managed differently to the companions. An obese donkey is at high risk of developing serious health problems.

Key to the formulation of management and dietary plans is awareness that the requirements of donkeys are very different to those of horses and ponies. Failure to do so can lead to disease and behavioural issues.

⚠ **ALERT**

The donkey is supremely adapted to survive on fodder which would generally be inadequate for horses and ponies.

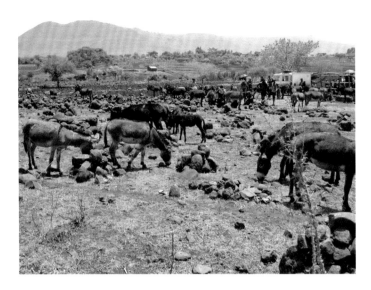

The donkey has evolved to live in semi-arid environments with only poor quality, sparse vegetation.

NUTRITIONAL REQUIREMENTS

The donkey should be fed a diet high in fibre and low in energy and nonstructural carbohydrates. The majority of the diet is best supplied using straws or stover (the leaves and stalks of field crops such as corn, maize or sorghum) and supplemented with a variable proportion of moderate quality hay and/or grazing depending on what is available locally.

Feeding recommendations are often extrapolated from horse nutrition. However, this will result in an overestimate of the nutrient requirements for maintenance and for work.

Energy requirements

Digestible energy requirements for maintenance in the donkey are often significantly overestimated.

Projects conducted in the UK and Mexico have established digestible energy (DE) and dry matter intake (DMI) requirements for maintenance of mature donkeys fed fibrous forages (barley straw or maize stover) supplemented with hay or grazing, and have investigated seasonal variability in these requirements.

Results suggest:

- Voluntary intake for donkeys on such diets is 1.3—1.7% daily of their bodyweight (bwt) in dry matter (DM) (2—2.5% recommended for ponies).

- For a 180kg donkey this equates to 2.5—3.1kg of DM per day.

- For maintenance, donkeys require between 80—95kJ DE/kg bwt/day.

- This is dependent upon the season (the lower value in each range is required when average daytime temperatures are higher than 18ºC).

➜ *See Appendix 7 for example diets for the mature, pregnant and lactating donkey.*

Companion and non-working donkeys require foodstuffs with low energy values so that they can eat enough to satisfy their natural appetite and satisfy the behavioural need to forage without becoming obese.

Working donkeys may require supplementary feeds, either due to the increased energy requirement or a lack of time to consume sufficient forage.

Supplementary feeding should focus on higher quality fibre sources such as grass hay, alfalfa or grazing. Where concentrates are required they should be low in cereal grain content in order to avoid related health problems.

Protein, vitamin and mineral requirements

⚠ **ALERT**

Additional protein may improve recovery time following surgery or injury or may be needed by young stock or pregnant or lactating female donkeys. Soya bean meal or alfalfa are excellent sources.

Studies to establish donkeys' requirements for protein, vitamins and minerals are limited. Research suggests:

- Protein requirements are significantly lower than those of horses and ponies.

- Crude protein (CP) requirements are 40g CP/100kg bwt/day. In practice, for most mature healthy donkeys, protein requirements tend to be satisfied once digestible energy (DE) requirements are satisfied.

- Provision of additional quality protein to donkeys recovering from surgery or injury may improve recovery times; protein deficiency may limit tissue repair. Soya bean meal or alfalfa are excellent sources of digestible protein for convalescent donkeys.

- Generally, appropriate levels of vitamins and minerals are similar to requirements for horses and ponies.

- Care must be taken to balance calcium and phosphorus and to ensure sufficient levels of vitamin supplementation to animals fed primarily on dried forages.

- Donkeys maintained on dried forages or being fed high levels of oil (greater than 100ml) may be at risk of vitamin E deficiency, which could increase the risk of equine degenerative myeloencephalopathy or equine motor neurone disease, although no evidence is available.

- The levels of vitamins and minerals recommended for horses and ponies represent an appropriate, optimal level of provision. However, The Donkey Sanctuary believes that donkeys are able to survive on vitamin and mineral levels lower than those recommended for horses and ponies.

- Provision of sodium chloride to donkeys working in hot environments may be beneficial. Salt should be provided *ad libitum*, it is not recommended that it is added to other feed products.

- Provision of adequate vitamins and minerals is best achieved by allowing daily access to fresh grazing with an equine mineral lick or vitamin and mineral supplement or balancer where possible.

THE NORMAL DIET

Donkeys thrive on fibrous forages with a low energy density. The most suitable way of providing a low energy diet is to offer straw where the cereal grain has been removed through harvesting (barley, oat or wheat) or stover (the leaves and stalks of field crops such as corn, maize or sorghum).

There may be a reluctance to feed straw to donkeys and mules due to concerns relating to colic and gastric ulcers. However, studies carried out in a large population of donkeys showed no increased risk of impaction colic or gastric ulceration associated with such feeding practices in donkeys with good dental health.

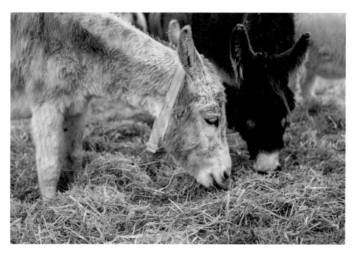

Straw will provide a suitable low energy diet.

It is important to:

- monitor donkeys with reduced mobility
- ensure that dental care is up to date
- ensure that intake is monitored regularly.

The donkey should also be provided with restricted grazing, hay or haylage. The proportions of such forages can be increased for animals struggling to maintain weight.

➔ *See Appendix 7 for example diets for the mature, pregnant and lactating donkey.*

Where pasture is sparse or of poor quality, and particularly in warmer arid climates, free access to grazing may provide most of the donkey's needs. However, donkeys fed solely on energy dense pasture often found in temperate climates may become obese or need to have their total dietary intake restricted to such an extent that they are at risk of developing gastric ulceration or stereotypies.

Consider the typical donkey behaviour traits when planning the diet:

- Donkeys form strong bonds and it is often essential to have the companion at least within sight, otherwise one or both animals may refuse to eat despite their hunger.

- Donkeys may 'sham eat' for considerable periods of time; the animal appears to mouth and swallow food or may simply nudge it but intake nothing. Such behaviour is often a sign of a serious illness and should be investigated promptly. Hyperlipaemia must always be considered.

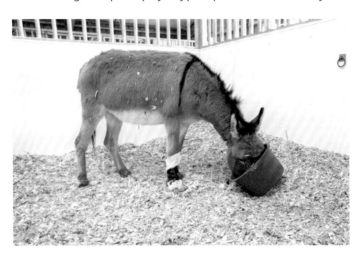

The donkey may look as though it is eating but may be sham eating (giving the impression of prehension, mastication and swallowing while actually ingesting very little).

- Donkeys generally tolerate the presence of others well and may be fed successfully in a group. However:

  - Dominant donkeys may bully other animals lower in the hierarchy and care should be taken to provide ample feeder space to prevent reduced intake by submissive animals.

  - Commonly donkeys are bullied at feed time by horses, ponies or mules, and may end up injured or unable to access enough feed to satisfy their requirements.

It is important to be aware that:

- Equine feedstuffs based upon cereals or containing high levels of molasses should be avoided. They have been shown to be risk factors for the development of gastric ulcers and laminitis in donkeys and other equids.

- The practice of intermittent 'meal' feeding is also to be discouraged. It is likely to produce peaks in insulin or increases in gastric pH. It has also been associated with hyperlipaemia, gastric ulcers and impaction colic in the donkey.

⚠ **ALERT**

Equine feedstuffs based upon cereal grains or containing high levels of molasses should be avoided.

The provision of an inappropriate diet can lead to the development of conditions such as laminitis, gastric ulceration, hyperlipaemia and fatty liver disease.

MONITORING THE DIET

Body condition scoring and monitoring of weight are an essential part of donkey husbandry.

> ⚠ **ALERT**
>
> **Body condition scoring for donkeys requires a different technique to that used in horses and ponies.**

Donkeys lay down fat stores in more localised areas and have a different body shape than horses and ponies, and therefore it is essential that different techniques are used for body scoring donkeys.

➡ *See Appendix 3 for a table showing guidelines for body scoring in the donkey.*

The donkey has an angular frame alongside a pendulous abdomen, and is often incorrectly described as 'pot bellied'. The pendulous abdomen may be due to increased retention of fibre within the gut and the related increased volume of the large intestine, abdominal fat, or in sedentary animals a slackness of the abdominal muscles.

When scoring donkeys it is essential to feel the animal. Donkeys can have thick coats, especially in winter or when suffering from Pituitary pars intermedia dysfunction (PPID), and appearances are often deceptive. Areas where fat is commonly deposited include the neck, shoulders, back, rump and the dorsal and lateral thorax.

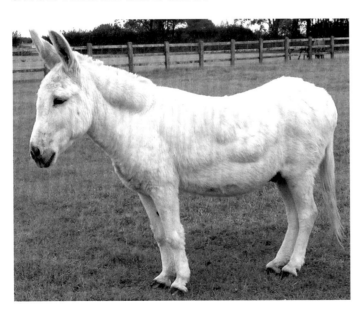

Obese donkey showing fat pads.

Donkeys frequently develop a fatty crest which may fall over to one side of the neck. Once in situ these deposits rarely disappear, even with dieting, and should be ignored in a mature animal that is in otherwise good condition. Fat pads are common on the buttocks and the dorsal and lateral thorax, and donkeys often carry significant abdominal fat (often up to 8cm, but increasing up to 14cm in the obese donkey). When such fat pads are longstanding they may become calcified and therefore extremely hard. They will never be lost through dieting and should be ignored when condition scoring.

Calcified fat pads are of clinical note; if the donkey is injured, a lack of blood supply to the area can promote the development of panniculitis, which may be difficult to treat.

FEEDING FOR COMMON CONDITIONS

The majority of donkeys manage very well on basic rations. However, there are cases which require specialist feeding.

Underweight donkeys

Before dietary changes can be made, a thorough clinical assessment should be carried out, including:

- observation of feeding behaviour and assessment of feeding and management practices (such as hobbling / tethering); these assessments are essential

- a thorough dental examination

- blood sampling to assess the overall health of the donkey, with particular attention to liver and kidney function, PPID and Equine Metabolic Syndrome (EMS)

- assessing the parasitic burden

- checking the workload and the availability of feedstuffs during working hours

- checking the level of preparation of feedstuffs; would products provided benefit from being chopped, rolled, cracked or soaked to provide ready access to nutrients?

Working donkeys unable to access adequate feedstuffs are prone to a poor body condition score. In addition such animals may have concurrent disease. Both working and companion donkeys with a low body condition score may have concurrent dental disease, liver disease or issues with companions; bullying or separation grief. A holistic approach to resolving all underlying causes is essential. When managing animals that require extra condition, it is important to encourage increased energy intake throughout the day by providing, for example, higher quantities of hay or a short-chopped fibre product.

Obesity

As in all species, obesity is a significant welfare problem and predisposes to a number of diseases.

Recent studies have shown that obese donkeys have higher insulin values, which are significantly associated with a history of laminitis. Obesity and associated hyperinsulinaemia may increase the risk of a donkey developing laminitis, particularly that associated with grazing.

Dietary management of obese donkeys is challenging and requires ongoing veterinary input.

Inappropriate diet is often compounded by lack of exercise, issues with companions; bullying or separation grief and EMS.

While obesity is uncommon in working donkeys, those that are worked infrequently or are kept for production purposes may also be at risk of obesity and related issues.

A management approach to the obese donkey should include:

- A dental check to ensure that the donkey can be given a diet based on straw or stover.

- An assessment of the donkey's ability to exercise.

- An appropriate blood sample.

➔ *See Chapter 7: Hyperlipaemia and the Endocrine System for more information on hyperlipaemia, PPID and EMS.*

Information from these checks will help to produce a plan for the obese donkey:

- Donkeys with high triglycerides (higher than 2.8 mmol/l) should have an exercise programme initiated before dietary changes are made. Once levels fall within the normal range, dietary changes may be introduced.

- Dietary management for obese or laminitic animals or those with EMS that have healthy teeth should focus on straw with very limited grazing in warm climates, and straw with limited hay when weather is cold (lower than 10°C). If there are concerns about deficiency, proprietary vitamin, mineral and protein supplements may be fed in small quantities.

Pasture management should be part of the plan:

- Restrict intake by strip grazing. A guide of less than 0.2 acre (less than 0.08 ha) per donkey of short cropped pasture is reasonable, and benefits from rotation, and no more than a total of 0.5 acres (0.2 ha) per donkey should be available.

- Evidence suggests that fructan levels in grass may only rarely be sufficient to trigger ration induced laminitis due to disrupted fermentation in the hind gut.

- High nonstructural carbohydrate (NSC) (simple sugars, starch and fructan) levels in grass may lead to increased insulin resistance and the development of endocrine related laminitis.

- Maintain a healthy grass sward as nonstructural carbohydrate levels can be high in lush grass but also in frosty grass and grass stressed by drought or overgrazing.

- Management by reduction of time at grazing has been shown to have little effect upon the total dietary intake of donkeys and may lead to them spending every minute at pasture eating rather than exercising and carrying out social behaviours. This may be followed by long periods of confinement which only exacerbates the issue.

In order to encourage donkeys to lose weight, they should be appropriately exercised wherever possible.

Donkeys should be condition scored and have their weight estimated monthly. Progress when dieting donkeys is slow, and perseverance is essential. It often takes weeks for the first weight to be lost. However, once this process begins, weight loss should be gradual. The aim should be to lose 2—3% of bodyweight monthly.

The inappetent donkey

Donkeys are particularly prone to developing hyperlipaemia.

➡ *See Chapter 7: Hyperlipaemia and the Endocrine System for more information.*

⚠ **ALERT**

A dull and inappetent donkey has a high risk of hyperlipaemia and is always a clinical emergency.

Donkeys with some voluntary appetite

Research has shown that inappetence or anorexia, often accompanied by dullness or lethargy, are the most frequent presenting signs when dealing with sick donkeys.

Many sick donkeys will maintain an appetite and should be given a diet similar to that normally provided. If hospitalised they may be provided with straw if this is what the donkey is accustomed to.

⚠ **ALERT**

Take caution must be exercised with patients on NSAIDs and with limited mobility when fed such diets.

When patients are prescribed NSAIDs caution must be exercised and frequent evaluation and recording of faecal output and gut sounds should be undertaken.

Nutritional management of sick donkeys often focuses upon the need to stimulate the donkey's appetite. However, although molasses and cereal grains can be used successfully in the short term, they can be detrimental in the long term.

Many donkeys can be tempted with fibrous equine feeds by adding tempters such as:

- mint cordial
- yeast extracts
- dried/fresh mint
- bananas, including the skin
- ginger, grated or in powder form
- carrots, apples, grated, juiced or chopped
- unmolassed beet pulp, soaked
- other locally available fruit or vegetables known to be safe for equines.

While nursing a sick donkey:

- Tempt the animal to eat from the hand, because large buckets are often refused.
- Do not underestimate the donkey's natural instinct as a browser, particularly in the case of sick animals.
- Donkeys that have shown no interest in food may be tempted to eat if led to a nearby hedgerow or scrub area to browse on brambles and herbs; this natural instinct can often be used successfully in the worst of cases.
- Ensure the sick donkey's companion is close by, even within a hospital setting.

A dental examination should be carried out. Blood samples should be used to assess the overall health of the donkey, paying particular attention to triglyceride concentration and parameters relating to liver and kidney function, PPID and EMS.

➡ *See Appendix 4 for the biochemical parameters for a donkey.*

Donkeys without voluntary appetite

When administering treatment by nasogastric tube or oral drenching, the potential for exacerbating or predisposing to hyperlipaemia through resultant stress must be balanced with the clinical needs of the patient.

When administering fluids by nasogastric tubing for more than a couple of days, provision of sufficient potassium should be ensured as it is rapidly excreted and insufficient levels may lead to ileus. Inclusion of 1g potassium chloride in every litre of fluids should be sufficient, alongside normal tubing preparations.

Patients should be fed with a fibre rich product, such as a ground instant oat breakfast cereal (for example Ready Brek). The addition of pre- and probiotics is beneficial. Consideration should be given to the administration of gastric protectants.

In hyperlipaemia cases parenteral nutrition should be considered and such treatment should begin promptly.

 See Chapter 7: Hyperlipaemia and the Endocrine System for more information on parenteral nutrition.

Dental disease

Dental disease is common in donkeys, particularly geriatrics, and this often leads to an inability to chew long fibre forages, causing gradual weight loss with associated depression and lethargy. In serious cases, dental pain can lead to a donkey becoming inappetent and predisposed to hyperlipaemia.

It is essential to replace long fibre forages with alternative fibre sources that can be easily chewed and digested. Short-chopped products designed for laminitic equines are suitable, and many of the low-energy products can be used to replace all fibre sources. Chopped fibre forages should be provided frequently throughout the day and be fed to dry matter intake (DMI) requirements. Although feeding of such products *ad libitum* may lead to gorging in the short term, intake is often self-regulating after a few weeks.

Donkeys that do not require such drastic changes in diet can be given small, frequent feeds of high fibre concentrates and unmolassed sugar beet pulp, alongside forage.

Laminitis

In the acute stages of laminitis it is essential to remove any contributory dietary issues. The donkey should be removed from pasture and given a high fibre, low nonstructural carbohydrate (NSC) diet.

Note that:

- It is essential to maintain fibre intake as starvation of the donkey is likely to result in hyperlipaemia.

- Straw may be fed but with decreased mobility checks must be maintained on gut motility and faecal output.

- A short-chopped forage with an NSC level of less than 10% is ideal to maintain the animal in the short term.

- Hay may be fed but be aware that NSC levels in some hay is high and may be inappropriate.

- Encourage water intake. Warmed water or water flavoured with small amounts of fruit juice or mint may be useful and provide enrichment.

- Haylage can be suitable but a high-fibre product with declared NSC content should be used. Sugar levels are often lower in haylage than hay due to fermentation.

- Sloppy feeds of unmolassed beet are useful to encourage water intake and assist with the administration of drugs.

Long-term management of the chronic laminitic is the same as that already described for obese animals.

Liver and kidney disease

Dietary management is a key component of a treatment plan for donkeys suffering from liver or kidney disease.

The donkey with liver disease needs a low protein diet resulting in reduced ammonia production. Such a diet, with less than 8% protein, can be met by grass, hay, straw and pasture. In addition:

- avoid alfalfa or cereal based feeds

- levels of fat within the diet should be controlled

- supplementary oil is discouraged

- short-chops, unmolassed beet pulp and high-fibre cubes are suitable where supplementary feeding is required.

Kidney disease patients should have a diet low in calcium and protein (less than 8%) and, where possible, should be maintained on hay and pasture. In addition:

- avoid legumes such as alfalfa and clover containing high levels of protein and calcium

- if required, extra energy can be supplied in the form of high oil supplements

- feed balancers designed for native ponies are also useful in such cases.

FEEDING IN PREGNANCY

Nutrient requirements for pregnancy and lactation in the donkey have yet to be established. The following guidelines are extrapolated from horse and pony data:

- In the final trimester, the female donkey will have a greater energy requirement, and it is important to supply quality protein, vitamins and minerals as the foal grows.

- In order to supply these nutrients, the energy density and quality of forages must be increased:

  - Gradually increase the hay portion of the diet until it constitutes the majority of the diet.

  - Use a supplement containing vitamins, minerals and protein, with low nonstructural carbohydrate (NSC) levels as designed for small ponies, at 75% of the levels recommended for ponies of a similar size.

  - If good quality hay is not available, supplementation with alfalfa or unmolassed beet pulp is useful.

- During pregnancy, the digestive tract capacity will decrease, which may lead to the female donkey being unable to satisfy the energy requirements of herself and the foal. This may leave her predisposed to hyperlipaemia and care should be taken to ensure energy requirements are met.

- A slight increase in condition before foaling is acceptable (body condition score 3.5) to allow for expected weight loss in the early stages of lactation.

- While lactating, the female donkey should receive adequate, good quality pasture and hay. Supplementation with vitamin and mineral products, chopped alfalfa or high fibre concentrates may also be indicated.

➔ *See Appendix 7 for example diets for the mature, pregnant and lactating donkey.*

- Hyperlipaemia is a concern in the lactating donkey. Owners should monitor appetite and provide adequate feed.

- The foal should be allowed to pick at the dam's feed in preparation for weaning. In general, donkey foals are weaned at approximately six months old.

> ⚠ **ALERT**
>
> It is advisable to monitor the foal's growth rate every two weeks during the lactation period.

- Foals should grow steadily and it is best practice to monitor the weight and condition of the foal every two weeks. If the rate of growth is too rapid, nutritional intake should be restricted, but with appropriate vitamin and mineral supplementation.

- If the foal is stunted, give appropriate supplementary feeding.

Expert advice should be sought in these situations.

🐎 MULES AND HINNIES

A diet based on fibrous forages and limited grazing is usually sufficient for the majority of mules.

Body condition scoring for mules requires a different technique to that used in horses and ponies.

Mules lie somewhere between the horse and donkey, with a rump that resembles that of a horse and a neck and lateral and dorsal thorax which stores fat like a donkey. These differences must be accounted for when condition scoring.

ℹ FURTHER INFORMATION

Factsheets, research and detailed information can be found online at:
thedonkeysanctuary.org.uk/for-professionals

Burden, F. (2012), Practical feeding and condition scoring for donkeys and mules. *Equine Veterinary Education*, 24: 589–596.

Lamoot, I., Callebaut, J., Demeulenaere, E., Vandenberghe, C. and Hoffman, M. (2005) Foraging behaviour of donkeys grazing in a coastal dune area in temperate climate conditions. *Applied Animal Behaviour Science*. 92 (1) 93 - 112.

Pearson, R.A., Archibald, R.F. and Muirhead, R.H. (2001) The effect of forage quality and level of feeding on digestibility and gastrointestinal transit time of oat straw and alfalfa given to ponies and donkeys. *British Journal of Nutrition*. 85. 599-606.

Wood, S.J., Smith, D.G., and Morris, C.J. (2005). 'Seasonal variation of digestible energy requirements of mature donkeys in the UK.' *Proceedings Equine Nutrition Conference*, Hanover, Germany. 1-2 October 2005. Pp 39-40.

APPENDICES

All of the following appendices are available for download in A4 format from our website at **thedonkeysanctuary.org.uk/for-professionals**

APPENDIX 1: THE CLINICAL EXAMINATION

Examination	Parameter	Units	Average	Range	Important points
Demeanour and behaviour *Observation* *History*	**A DULL DONKEY IS VERY LIKELY TO BE SERIOUSLY ILL. TREAT AS AN EMERGENCY.**				Very subtle changes in behaviour may indicate severe disease. A dull donkey usually indicates stress or pain (e.g. colic, hyperlipaemia, laminitis, dental disease, liver disease). Observe mobility; signs of lameness or increased recumbency.
Body condition appetite *Body score* *Skin*	**Weight** Important for medication See Appendices 2 and 3 for weight estimator and body scoring chart.	Kg	180	90-400	Watch for "sham" eating (pretending to eat) The thick hair coat can hide skin conditions and mask a poor body score: use a donkey specific body score chart. Palpate and check for skin conditions, lumps, parasites etc. 180 is average for a UK donkey.
Temperature	Adult donkey	°C °F	37.1 98.8	36.5-37.8 97.2-100	Newborn foal - 37.5-38.5°C, 99.5-101.3°F
	Young donkey	°C °F	37.6 99.6	36.2-38.9 97-102	
Cardiac auscultation and pulse rate	Adult donkey	Beats per minute	44	36-52	>52 indicates stress or pain. >70 could indicate severe pain or hypovolaemic shock without pain. Pulse quality may be less affected by dehydration and fluid loss in the donkey.
	Young donkey Newborn foal		60	40-80 80-120	
Respiratory tract auscultation and respiratory rate	Adult donkey	Breaths per minute	20	12-28	Consider the use of a re-breathing bag to accentuate subtle lung sounds, especially in obese donkeys where fat deposits muffle sounds. The donkey has an insensitive cough reflex. The respiratory rate decreases in the newborn foal after 12 hours.
	Young donkey		28	16-48	
	Newborn foal After 12 hours			60-80 30-40	
Mucous membranes colour *Texture e.g. moist/tacky* *Capillary refill time*	Capillary refill time	Seconds	1.5	1-2.5	Capilliary refill time may remain close to normal despite fluid loss or dehydration.
Abdominal auscultation	Auscultation of borborgymi				Both mixing and propulsive contractions should be auscultated and sounds should be present in all 4 quarters of the abdomen, where size allows delineation.
Examination of the oral cavity	An essential part of any clinical examination in the donkey.				The use of an oral speculum is essential as the narrow mandibular arcade makes visualisation more challenging.
Ocular examination					Note the different location of the nasal opening of the nasolacrimal duct in the donkey.
Rectal examination					Can be safely performed in most donkeys with care and lubrication. A spasmolytic can be used.
Peritoneal tap					A peritoneal tap can be difficult because of adipose deposits along ventral body wall (be aware that fat may be up to 14cm in depth in obese donkeys).
Ultrasound					Subcutaneous fat may obscure detail from ultrasound imaging.
Blood sample *Haemotology, biochemistry and screen for hyperlipaemia*	Triglycerides See appendix 4 for other parameters.	mmol/l	1.4	0.6-2.8	>2.8 mmol/l indicates mild hyperlipaemia. >8 mmol/l indicates moderate disease with increased mortality rates. >15mmol/l indicates severe disease with significantly increased mortality rates.

APPENDIX 2: DONKEY WEIGHT ESTIMATOR

To estimate a donkey's weight using the diagram below mark the height and heart girth measurements on the correct axis. Then draw a line between the two. The donkey's weight is indicated by where the line crosses the weight axis. For example, a donkey 104cm tall (a) and with a heart girth 122cm (b) should weigh 181kg (c).

Donkey weight estimator

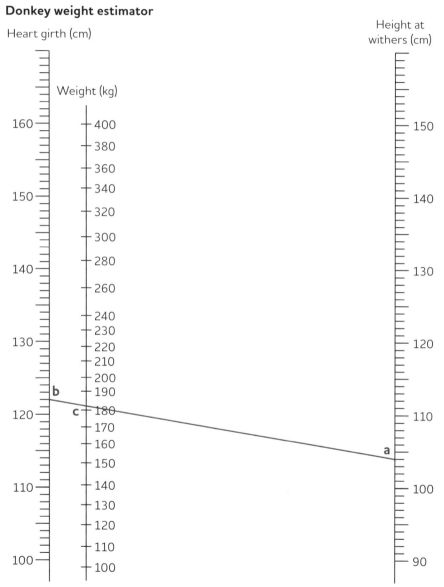

Whilst the weight estimator is an effective tool to estimate weight it's accuracy cannot be guaranteed.

Weight estimation table for donkeys under 2 years

Heart Girth (cm)	75	76	77	78	79	80	81	82	83	84	85	86	87	88	89	90	91	92	93	94	95	96	97	98	99	100
Weight (kg)	46	47	49	51	53	55	57	59	61	63	65	67	69	71	74	76	78	81	83	86	88	91	94	96	99	102

APPENDIX 3: BODY SCORING

Donkey body condition score chart

Condition Score	Neck and shoulders	Withers	Ribs and belly	Back and loins	Hindquarters
1. Poor	Neck thin, all bones easily felt. Neck meets shoulder abruptly, shoulder bones felt easily, angular.	Dorsal spine of withers Prominent and easily felt.	Ribs can be seen from a distance and felt with ease. Belly tucked up.	Backbone prominent, can feel dorsal and transverse processes easily.	Hip bones visible and felt easily (hock and pin bones). Little muscle cover. May be cavity under tail.
2. Moderate	Some muscle development overlying bones. Slight step where neck meets shoulders.	Some cover over dorsal withers, spinous processes felt but not prominent.	Ribs not visible but can be felt with ease.	Dorsal and transverse processes felt with light pressure. Poor muscle development either side midline.	Poor muscle cover on hindquarters, hipbones felt with ease.
3. Ideal	Good muscle development, bones felt under light cover of muscle/fat. Neck flows smoothly into shoulder, which is rounded.	Good cover of muscle/fat over dorsal spinous processes withers flow smoothly into back.	Ribs just covered by light layer of fat/muscle, ribs can be felt with light pressure. Belly firm with good muscle tone and flattish outline.	Cannot feel individual spinous or transverse processes. Muscle development either side of midline is good.	Good muscle cover in hindquarters, hipbones rounded in appearance, can be felt with light pressure.
4. Fat	Neck thick, crest hard, shoulder covered in even fat layer.	Withers broad, bones felt with firm pressure.	Ribs dorsally only felt with firm pressure, ventral ribs may be felt more easily. Belly over developed.	Can only feel dorsal and transverse processes with firm pressure. Slight crease along midline.	Hindquarters rounded, bones felt only with firm pressure. Fat deposits evenly placed.
5. Obese	Neck thick, crest bulging with fat and may fall to one side. Shoulder rounded and bulging with fat.	Withers broad, unable to feel bones.	Large, often uneven fat deposits covering dorsal and possibly ventral aspect of ribs. Ribs not palpable. Belly pendulous in depth and width.	Back broad, unable to feel spinous or transverse processes. Deep crease along midline bulging fat either side.	Cannot feel hipbones, fat may overhang either side of tail head, fat often uneven and bulging.

APPENDIX 4: PARAMETERS: BIOCHEMISTRY AND HAEMATOLOGY

Parameters for an adult donkey.

Haematology			
	Result	Ave	Range
RBC	1012/l	5.5	(4.4 – 7.1)
PCV	%	33	(27 – 42)
Hb	g/dl	11.0	(8.9 – 14.7)
MCH	pg	20.6	(17.6 – 23.1)
MCHC	g/dl	34	(31 – 37)
MCV	fl	60	(53 – 67)
WBC	109/l	10	(6.2 – 15)
NEU%	%	38.3	(23 – 59)
NEU T	109/l	3.7	(2.4 – 6.3)
EOS%	%	4.0	(0.9 – 9.1)
EOS T	109/l	0.4	(0.1 – 0.9)
BAS%	%	0.05	(0 – 0.5)
BAS T	109/l	0	(0 – 0.07)
LYM%	%	54	(34 – 69)
LYM T	109/l	5.5	(2.2 – 9.6)
MON%	%	3.0	(0.5 – 7.5)
MON T	109/l	0.3	(0 – 0.75)
Platelets	109/l	201	(95 – 384)
RDW	%	18.3	(16.1 – 22)

Biochemistry			
	Result	Ave	Range
Trig	mmol/l	1.4	(0.6 – 2.8)
CPK	u/l	208	(128 – 525)
AST	u/l	362	(238 – 536)
GGT	u/l	24	(14 – 69)
GLDH	u/l	2.5	(1.2 – 8.2)
ALP	u/l	152	(98 – 252)
Bile acids	µmol/l	10	(2.6 – 18.6)
Tbil	µmol/l	1.6	(0.1 – 3.7)
TP	g/l	65	(58 – 76)
Alb	g/l	26	(22 – 32)
Glob	g/l	38	(32 – 48)
Creat	µmol/l	87	(53 – 118)
Urea	mmol/l	3.2	(1.5 – 5.2)
Amylase	u/l	4	(1 – 10.6)
Lipase	u/l	12.9	(7.8 – 27.3)
Glucose	mmol/l	4.43	(3.9 – 4.7)
Calcium	mmol/l	3	(2.2 – 3.4)
Na	mmol/l	133	(128 – 138)
K	mmol/l	4.3	(3.2 – 5.1)
Cl	mmol/l	102	(96 – 106)
Chol	mmol/l	2.0	(1.4 – 2.9)

Clotting Factors		
	Result	Range
Fibrinogen	g/l	(0.6 – 2.6)
Prothromb	seconds	(8.9 – 14.5)

APPENDIX 5: MONITORING YOUR DONKEY'S QUALITY OF LIFE

Name of donkey:

Date:

Heart girth measurement (refer to nomogram):

Feeding	Yes	No	Comments
Change in diet			
Enthusiastic to eat			
Dropping food			
Choking on food			
Drooling			
Behaviour	**Yes**	**No**	**Comments**
Alert (frequently moving ears or is head and ear carriage lower)			
Responsive			
Interacting with friends			
Lying down more			
Lying down less			
Difficulty in getting up			
Difficulty getting down			
Enjoying a daily roll			
Locomotion	**Yes**	**No**	**Comments**
Walking and trotting easily			
Turning without difficulty			
Hooves same shape and size			
Walking as much as before			
A bit slower/pottery/taking shorter strides			
Using all of the paddock			
Enjoying walks			
Breathing	**Yes**	**No**	**Comments**
Breathing with ease			
Carrying out normal activities without getting out of breath or exhibiting flared nostrils			
Laboured or noisy breathing			
General	**Yes**	**No**	**Comments**
Any lumps			
Bad breath			
Any eye discharge			
Any nasal discharge			
Passing faeces normally			
Wounds on hocks/knees - indicates difficulty rising			

For more information please watch the video Growing Old Gracefully online:
thedonkeysanctuary.org.uk/for-professionals

APPENDIX 6: VETERINARY RECORD OF ASSESSMENT FOR QUALITY OF LIFE

Name of animal:	Name of owner:
Age/year of birth:	Discussion with owner:

Major condition:

QOL end points:

☐ Loss of condition despite increased feed
☐ Recurrence of laminitis
☐ Lameness on maintenance dose NSAID
☐ Anorexia, dullness or colic
☐ Blindness causing distress

Minor condition(s):	Any further comments:

Date	Weight kg	Condition Score	Feed	Appetite	Blood Results	Demeanour	Medicines and doses	Dental Condition	Skin condition	Use of rug	Movement and Feet	Progress of condition

APPENDIX 7: EXAMPLE DIETS: FOR THE MATURE, PREGNANT AND LACTATING DONKEY

Mature donkeys fed on fibrous forages:

Donkey weight	MJ, DE/day	Daily DMI requirement	Suggested diet
180 kg donkey maintenance (summer)	14.4	2.4 kg	2.1 kg barley straw (5 MJ DE/kg DM) + limited grazing or + 0.5 kg moderate hay (8 MJ DE/kg DM)
180 kg donkey maintenance (winter)	17.1	3.1 kg	3 kg barley straw (5 MJ DE/kg DM) + 0.4 kg moderate hay (8 MJ DE/kg DM)
Dieting donkey goal weight 180 kg (summer)	13	2.4 kg	2.2 kg barley straw (5 MJ DE/kg DM) + very limited grazing or + 0.2 kg moderate hay (8 MJ DE/kg DM) + forage balancer
Dieting donkey goal weight 180 kg (winter)	15.5	3.1 kg	3.1 kg barley straw (5 MJ DE/kg DM) + very limited grazing or + forage balancer
180 kg donkey (aged) with dental disease (summer)	14.4–15	2.4 kg	2.4 kg short chop hay replacer (7.3 MJ DE/kg DM assuming 85% DM) e.g. forage balancer
180 kg donkey (aged) with dental disease (winter)	17.1–18	3.1 kg	2.9 kg short chop hay replacer (7.3 MJ DE/kg DM assuming 85% DM) e.g. forage balancer

Pregnant donkeys in the final 3 months of pregnancy:

Donkey weight	MJ, DE/day	Daily DMI requirement	Suggested diet
180 kg - 9 months gestation (summer)	16.7	2–2.4 kg	1.1 kg barley straw (5 MJ DE/kg DM) + grazing and high protein balancer or + 1.3 kg moderate hay (8.5 MJ DE/kg DM) and high protein balancer
180 kg - 10 months gestation (summer)	17.4	2–2.4 kg	0.4 kg barley straw (5 MJ DE/kg DM) + 1.8 kg moderate hay (8.5 MJ DE/kg DM) + high protein balancer
180 kg - 11 months gestation (summer)	18.6	2–2.4 kg	2.2 kg moderate hay (8.5 MJ DE/kg DM) + high protein balancer + grazing If hay is not managed supplement with high fibre cubes, alfalfa chop or unmolassed sugar beet
180 kg - 9 months gestation (winter)	19.8	2.5–3.1 kg	1 kg barley straw (5 MJ DE/kg DM) 1.7 kg moderate hay (8.5 MJ DE/kg DM) + high protein balancer
180 kg - 10 months gestation (winter)	20.7	2.5–3.1 kg	2.2 kg moderate hay (8.5 MJ DE/kg DM) 0.4 kg barley straw (5 MJ DE/kg DM) + high protein balancer
180 kg - 11 months gestation (winter)	22.1	2.5–3 kg	2.5 kg moderate hay (8.5 MJ DE/kg DM) + 200 g alfalfa chop (9 MJ DE/kg DM) + high protein balancer

Lactating donkeys:

Donkey weight	MJ, DE/day	Daily DMI requirement	Suggested diet
180 kg lactation 1st month (summer)	27.5	2.4–3 kg	2.4 kg good hay (9 MJ DE/kg DM) + grazing and high protein balancer or 0.3 kg alfalfa oil chop (11.2 MJ DE/kg DM) and high protein balancer
180 kg lactation 2nd month (summer)	27.3	2.4–3 kg	2.6 kg good hay (9 MJ DE/kg DM) + grazing and high protein balancer or 0.2 kg alfalfa oil chop (11.2 MJ DE/kg DM) and high protein balancer
180 kg lactation 3rd month (summer)	26.5	2.4–3 kg	2.6 kg good hay (9 MJ DE/kg DM) + grazing and high protein balancer or 0.15 kg alfalfa oil chop (11.2 MJ DE/kg DM) and high protein balancer
180 kg lactation 4th month (summer)	25.5	2.4–3 kg	2.6 kg good hay (9 MJ DE/kg DM) + grazing and high protein balancer or 0.1 kg alfalfa oil chop (11.2 MJ DE/kg DM) and high protein balancer
180 kg lactation 5th month (summer)	24.5	2.4–3 kg	2.5 kg good hay (9 MJ DE/kg DM) + grazing and high protein balancer or 0.1 kg alfalfa oil chop (11.2 MJ DE/kg DM) and high protein balancer
180 kg lactation 6th month (summer)	23.6	2.4–3 kg	2.4 kg good hay (9 MJ DE/kg DM) + grazing and high protein balancer
180 kg lactation 1st month (winter)	30.2	2.7–3.1 kg	3 kg good hay (9 MJ DE/kg DM) + grazing and high protein balancer or 0.3 kg alfalfa oil chop (11.2 MJ DE/kg DM) and high protein balancer
180 kg lactation 2nd month (winter)	30	2.7–3.1 kg	3 kg good hay (9 MJ DE/kg DM) + grazing and high protein balancer or 0.2 kg alfalfa oil chop (11.2 MJ DE/kg DM) and high protein balancer
180 kg lactation 3rd month (winter)	29.2	2.7–3.1 kg	3 kg good hay (9 MJ DE/kg DM) + grazing and high protein balancer or 0.15 kg alfalfa oil chop (11.2 MJ DE/kg DM) and high protein balancer
180 kg lactation 4th month (winter)	28.2	2.7–3.1 kg	3 kg good hay (9 MJ DE/kg DM) + grazing and high protein balancer or 0.1 kg alfalfa oil chop (11.2 MJ DE/kg DM) and high protein balancer
180 kg lactation 5th month (winter)	27.2	2.7–3.1 kg	2.8 kg good hay (9 MJ DE/kg DM) + grazing and high protein balancer or 0.1 kg alfalfa oil chop (11.2 MJ DE/kg DM) and high protein balancer
180 kg lactation 6th month (winter)	26.3	2.4–3 kg	2.6 kg good hay (9 MJ DE/kg DM) grazing + high protein balancer

The table includes estimated dry matter intakes and practical dietary recommendations. DE values assume a dry matter content of 90% unless otherwise stated, foodstuffs such as haylage should be evaluated for DE levels per kg as fed and if unsure forage analysis is recommended.

Forage balancer refers to a concentrated pellet vitamin, mineral and protein supplement which does not act as a significant source of energy and which is designed to balance a forage only diet.

High protein balancer – as above but with a higher protein specification which is more suited to pregnant/lactating/growing donkeys.

INDEX